Where Nurse's Shoes Walk:

A Nurse's Journey

by

Mary Lu Gerke Ph.D.

DORRANCE PUBLISHING CO

The contents of this work, including, but not limited to, the accuracy of events, people, and places depicted; opinions expressed; permission to use previously published materials included; and any advice given or actions advocated are solely the responsibility of the author, who assumes all liability for said work and indemnifies the publisher against any claims stemming from publication of the work.

All Rights Reserved
Copyright © 2023 by Mary Lu Gerke Ph.D.

No part of this book may be reproduced or transmitted, downloaded, distributed, reverse engineered, or stored in or introduced into any information storage and retrieval system, in any form or by any means, including photocopying and recording, whether electronic or mechanical, now known or hereinafter invented without permission in writing from the publisher.

Dorrance Publishing Co
585 Alpha Drive
Pittsburgh, PA 15238
Visit our website at www.dorrancebookstore.com

ISBN: 979-8-89027-288-1
eISBN: 979-8-89027-786-2

Dedication

To God, family, and friends who supported my nursing journey. Step by step, you were at my side.
Thank you.

Contents

Dedication..iii
Preface..ix
Why?...xi
Chapter One – The First Step, The Call.........................1
   Novice..2
   Working Nights..4
Chapter Two – Next Steps...7
   Diversity...7
   Crying with the family..9
Chapter Three – Urban Walking.................................13
   Walking Through the Storm.................................14
   Wounded Healer..16
Chapter Four – Next Step Nurse Educator 21
Chapter Five – Walking and Living the Dream..........27
   Leading Nurses Like a Shepherd..........................27
   Know the Condition of Your Flock 30
   Discover the Shape of Your Sheep 31
   Help Your Sheep Identify with You......................34
   The Staff of Direction – Responsibility to
   Direct People..35
   The Rod of Correction - Responsibility to
   Correct People..37
   The Heart of the Shepherd...................................40
   Walking in the Shoes of Patients and Family......41
   Comforting the Dying 43

Listening to Messages from Angels 45
Captain of the Ship 50
Chapter Six – If Not You, Who? 53
Patients and Families Come First! 54
Help me, Help you! 57
Mom – The Promise 61
Moving On 65
Chapter Seven – Traveling and Discovering New Path Executive Leadership – Vice President of Regional Services..67
Rural Patient Care 68
Closing and Opening 71
Chapter Eight – Giant Steps 75
Vice President of Nursing, Education and Research Assessment of Practicing Nurses 75
Statement from Nurses 77
Contemporary Nursing Practice Implementation 79
Celebration of Nurses 81
Western Campus of Nursing 85
Nursing Research 86
Chapter Nine – Unlikely Steps 89
Dean of Nursing 89
Assessment – Know the condition of the flock...91
Implementing Change – The Staff of Direction ..97
Need for Transitions – The Rod of Correction ...98
Chapter 10 – Muse 105
Retirement – Into the Woods 105

Principles and Themes of My Journey 106
Conclusion – A Time for Everything 109
Resources 110
Biographical Sketch...111

Preface

There is a whimper in the hallways of hospitals, clinics, nursing homes, and all health care facilities that serve patients, even patients in their home. Do you hear the whimper? It is the crying of a lost child. The lost child is the soul essence of nursing. Only lost, the child is still here and hopefully can be found. The question is, who will find the child, the essence of nursing, and will it be soon enough?

Nurses across the country and perhaps the world are asking themselves, "What happened? How did we get to the point where the patient is not a unique individual but a number on the spreadsheet of the budget?" Has, "the patient always comes first no matter what," gone away? Nurses have a responsibility to make sure that the patient's priorities are the priorities. Some want to give excuses to this dilemma. It's the nursing shortage. Others blame the cost of healthcare and the business of healthcare. Perhaps these are contributing factors, but I feel this is not getting to the core of what has and is happening. The issues of shortages, reimbursement, the aging workforce, gender diversity, and the numerous excuses we use to cover the ugly problem need to be addressed by nurses.

Nursing is a "calling" and I am driven to write this book about finding our way back to soul and essence of nursing: The sacred ground of the patient-nurse relationship.

When we walk into the healthcare facility, we enter the sacred grounds of human interactions. People dealing with special moments in their lives: birth, diagnosis of chronic diseases, terminal illnesses, traumatic injuries, surgical repairs, and death. Nurses are granted a special blessing to share in these moments. David Whyte in one of his lectures speaks about Moses' mountain experience during the "burning bush" episode in his life. He says, "Moses is reminded by God that he needs to take off his shoes because he (Moses) is standing on Holy ground. Moses looks down and realizes that this indeed is Holy ground, and he has always been standing on Holy ground, he just wasn't aware of it." I want this book to bring awareness to nurses, physicians, administrators, and the general public that the Holy or Sacred ground nurses and healthcare personnel stand on every day. The sacred or holy ground is the relationship and shared events we have with mankind. This is a gift. It is a great "calling" and privilege to serve and participate in the life events of each patient. At this time in the history of the profession of nursing, nurses need to look down on and reflect on the sacred ground we walk. I believe we have just lost awareness of this phenomenon. We have been too busy looking ahead, worrying about being respected by other professions and not bathing in the awareness of the present, the gift of walking with each patient and family on their sacred journey of life. This book focuses on the independent, autonomous work of the professional registered nurse (RN). The work of educating, care planning with the patient and family, promoting comfort, self-care, stress-reduction, and coping with illness and death. For those who are seeking a path for giving and receiving blessings and joy, nursing is a wonderful choice as demonstrated in the exemplars and stories in this book.

Why?

A patient lay dying, the nurse raised her eyes to the heavens,

A tear ran down her cheek, she asked the Lord, "Why?"

God answered her in a consoling, teaching way, saying,

"My child, you needed today, a gift of sharing your love and caring."

A nurse exhausted and frustrated with a confused, combative patient,

Raised her eyes to heaven, and asked the Lord, "Why?"

God answered her with gentle kindness, saying,

"My child, today you needed a gift to help you learn patience."

A nurse helped deliver a healthy baby and placed the crying wonder in her mother's arms.

She wondered why she was given the blessing to witness this miracle and she asked the Lord, "Why?"

The Lord pleased with her gratitude responded,

"You are given blessing to lighten your load and the load of your friends and family.

Share this wonder and happiness with them."

A nurse, after contacting several physicians to obtain an order for a patient,

Raised her eyes to heaven and asked the Lord, "Why?"

God answered with a smile, saying,

"You needed to strengthen your spirit of persistence."

A nurse debrided, cleansed, and dressed a gaping wound for the fourth time on her shift.

She raised her eyes to heaven and asked the Lord, why would the wound not heal?

God answered gently, "My child, you are trying to heal the flesh,

Your work for this patient is to heal his spirit."

A young nurse manager finished a conversation with an angry staff nurse.

Unable to help her understand why there were not

more staff to help on her unit.

She raised her eyes to the heavens and asked the Lord, "Why?"

God responded, **a tear fell from His eye,** "My child, many are called, few are answering the call to serve." He paused and asked, **"Why?"**

Mary Lu Gerke, RN, Ph.D.

Chapter One
The First Step, The Call

How do we discern what our purpose on earth is according to God's will? Some are blessed and know without a doubt what their path is. But most struggle to figure out what their profession or path should be. I believe God can help. All we really have to do is ask. God is the way, the truth, and the life. So, when we are in times of stress or making decisions, it would be wise to ask for the guidance of God.

If you choose nursing, you will discover many blessings and struggles. Nursing is a complex and diverse field of practice. The work of a professional nurse (RN) includes functions that are regulated through licensure, some functions require collaboration and cooperation with other healthcare disciplines. Some functions of the nurse are considered exclusive or independent, being autonomously performed at the nurse's discretion, such as educating patients and families, developing plans with the patient and family to promote comfort, self-care, stress-reduction, and coping with illness and death.

You also learn the importance of the healthcare team. The nursing functions of teamwork are defined as interdependent or shared with other healthcare disciplines or delegated to non-nursing personnel under the supervision of the nurse. Examples include ambulating patients, hygiene care, weighing patients, and preparing patients for discharge.

There are dependent functions. These are functions ordered by the physician like medication delivery, treatments and insertion of tubes, intravenous infusion, and use of mechanical intervention. With those in mind, let's start the journey of where white shoes walk in the profession of nursing.

Novice

I always knew I was supposed to be a nurse. What I didn't know was how God would help me in the practice of nursing. At first as novices, we don't know or don't use the great power of God. We learn, one day at a time, one experience at a time how to tap into the energy and spirit of God. How do we tap into this spirit? We can utilize the spirit of God in all situations by being attentive to signs. The signs and messages come from our surroundings, people who come into our life or purely listening. Throughout my career, I learned that the impossible became possible. When I didn't think I could make things happen, there often were people or incidents to make the way clear. I started to believe that the hospital was sacred ground. A place where there were people experiencing joy; like birth or recovery from illness and pain; like severe injuries and death.

I didn't learn to appreciate the power of trusting in God at first. But after reflecting on situations at the end of the day; I soon realized that there was a power much greater than man. Man is or can be instrumental in people's life.

I graduated from a Bachelor of Science in Nursing program in 1974. I remember my first day like it was yesterday. I hardly slept the night before my first day. I woke up early and put on my white uniform and white shoes for the first time as a registered nurse. I entered the conference room of the unit I was assigned to. The room was filled with smoke. Smoking was allowed at that time. The night shift charge nurse gave the report to the day charge nurse (the head nurse). The unit had forty beds. A large cardiac – medical unit. We all were assigned five or six patients. The report included information on each patient's condition, vital signs, and how their night had been. I listened attentively to information about my patients and wrote down the activities I would need to do for each patient. At the end of the report, we went to set up morning medications for each patient. There was no unit dose system at that time, so you had to take each medication from a general container and put in medication cups for each patient. Intermuscular medications needed to be mixed before drawing the medication up into a syringe. The medications were powder, and we would mix them with sterile water and draw them up in a syringe.

Each medication had a medication card with the patient's name, room, and of course the medication. Then we started distributing the medication.

One of the first areas nurses learn is how to communicate with patients and families. Entering the patient rooms, I greeted each patient and let them know my name and that I would be their nurse for the shift. I learned quickly that casual conversation should be focused on the patient and family. I would ask them how they were feeling, what had taken them to the hospital, and if they needed anything before I gave them their medications. I took each patient's blood pressure, pulse, and temperature, recording them in their chart. Before computerization, all information was manually written. This could be time-consuming but critical.

The best time to get to know the patient was during their bath and morning care. I would ask them about their life and family. Things like where they came from, what they did for a living, and their plans for recovery.

Most patients could have some type of breakfast. We sat the patient up and made sure they were able to eat and drink their breakfast. I discovered that the more you could put the patient at ease, the more they would be willing to eat and drink.

Working Nights

I was orientated to all three shifts. But as a new graduate,

I worked primarily the night shift. I didn't realize until later in my practice years how very important each experience would have on my future roles and practice.

The night shift was a special time to experience quiet moments in the usually hectic activities of the day and PM shifts. One night, I was doing my patients' rounds and walked into an elderly patient's room. He was not breathing well, so I stayed in the room for a while. The man grabbed my hand and asked if I would stay. The unit was quiet, so I was able to stay with him.

He said, "I know I don't have much more time. I just don't want to die alone."

I asked if he wanted me to call his relatives. He said he had very few relatives and they all were estranged.

"Well then," I said with a smile, "I will stay." I sat with him, and he gently fell asleep.

But soon his breathing slowed down and when I took his pulse it was also very slow. After about a half hour, his breathing stopped as well as his heartbeat. He was a "do not resuscitate" patient therefore no emergency intervention was necessary. The room seemed to be filled with an aura. A light cast across the bed and a feeling of peace was all around me. Some would say this was my imagination, but I believe that the angels were there to take him home. I learned from this experience; the patients know their condition better than any diagnostics. He knew he was dying. And I learned that being with a dying patient is a great blessing. A gift. Just like being present at a birth is a blessing, being present at a death is also a blessing.

As I learned nursing one day at a time, I became more and more in love with the caring of people.

Chapter Two
Next Steps

Being a novice teaches us the basic work and general care of the patients but once I accomplished that I was ready for the next steps on my path. I wouldn't have called myself an expert but felt confident to take the next step. What I soon discovered was that every time I took the next step, I became a novice again. There were open positions in the intensive care department. I was qualified to work in the intensive care unit and applied for a position. It was a small five-bed unit. The intensity of the patients was average. The unit was mostly medical patients with heart disease or other medical problems. I was exposed to patients in critical condition and learned the importance of monitoring and intervening in their care.

Diversity

On a weekend shift, I was assigned to a patient with esophageal varies. This condition exhibits bleeding coming from the esophagus caused by vessels in the esophagus that had ulcerated and started to bleed. The treatment for these patients at that time was to put a tube down their esophagus and put iced water down the tube and pull the water back out. Repeating this would cause the bleeding to stop. With this patient, the procedure did not work and he kept throwing up and profusely bleeding. The physician was called and came to see the patient. He said that the patient needed to be given blood. So, I prepared to infuse blood. However, giving blood had to be consented by the patient. The patient was a Jehovah's Witness. This religion did not allow people to receive blood infusions. We were left with only giving the patient intravenous fluids to support dehydration but without replacing the blood loss, he would not be able to survive. He would not survive surgery or any intervention without replacing his blood loss. The patient and family were given the prognosis and options. They continued to not have blood given. It was a difficult shift. I tried every explanation of the situation I could. But their religion was their decision maker. He soon lost consciousness and was near death when my shift ended.

I went home in an exhausted and stressed mood. I couldn't get him out of my mind. The solution for this situation was simply to give life-saving blood. I was sitting at my kitchen table when the doorbell rang. I went to the door and there was a representative of the Jehovah's Witness community. The elderly man started yelling at me and saying we had killed his friend and neighbor. I listened but decided not to argue and said I was so sorry. We had followed their wishes and there was nothing else we could do. After a few minutes, he left. I hoped and prayed that if yelling at me would make him feel better, that was good. I learned from experience that sometimes, no matter what we wanted to do, we had to follow the wishes of the patient and family. Little did I know how often I would experience these situations.

The time of being a novice was so important to the path that lay ahead. I kept a diary of every patient. This helped me reflect on my learnings. I encourage new graduates and novices of the profession to keep a diary for reflection and learning.

Crying with the family

The next year we were able to open a new intensive care unit. This unit was a twelve-bed unit with much larger rooms and state-of-the-art monitoring. Most of the rooms had windows which allowed some natural daylight to flow into the rooms. The environment was exciting to work in. The team of nursing colleagues I worked with taught me a great deal. Soon I was feeling comfortable and able to meet the most critical needs of our patients.

One morning as we finished the report, the emergency room called and said they were bringing a patient to the unit. He was a twenty-three-year-old white male who had an accident. He had been cutting trees down and a tree had fallen on him injuring his head, neck, and back. When they brought him, he was conscious and although in severe pain, he was able to communicate. His mother was with him. We made her comfortable in a chair in the room as we transferred her son into the ICU bed.

After hooking up the monitors and infusion tubes, we did the initial vital signs. All was going well. Suddenly, his monitor showed he was not breathing well and soon went in a heart arrythmia that called for emergency intervention. We called a "Code Blue". The physician, certified registered anesthetist (CRNA), respiratory staff, and other nurses responded. We started cardiac percussions and respirations (CPR) for the young man. The CRNA tried to insert an endotracheal tube, but he was having difficulty. I called the MD anesthesiologist. He also was unable to get the ET tube in the patient. We continued to deliver respirations but without better support, the patient was going to die. There was an attempt to perform a tracheotomy (an airway in the neck) but as the doctor soon found out the trachea itself had received damage and the swelling had closed off the patient's airway. The mother remained in the room during all of this work. The doctor said there was nothing more we could do.

The mother went to the bottom of her son's bed and started crying and screaming, "No, no, he cannot die. What will I do without him."

There wasn't a dry eye in the room. We all were crying. I put my arms around the mom and cried with her. I called the chaplain and stayed with her while we prayed for her son.

My reflection and learning on this experience was

the importance of being at the family's side. Crying with them and consoling them as best you can. Some nurses believe that nurses should not cry or show emotion. I can't disagree more.

I believe that after three years I had walked the path of novice and beginner. I felt I had experienced many events and learned a great deal. I was now ready to learn and do more. But I didn't think I could get that experience in this intensive care unit. I wanted to experience an intensive care unit that delivered care to open heart patients and critical trauma patients.

So, I started looking and found an intensive care unit in a metropolitan city in the Midwest. Leaving my colleagues and family was hard. I learned that when you walk down the path, you have to say good-bye, but you never lose friends and experiences.

Chapter Three
Urban Walking

The hospital was a large 500-bed hospital, located in a suburb of a metropolitan city in the Midwest. I interviewed for a position in the intensive care unit. I packed up my few belongings and headed out on a new adventure. Little did I know how much I would learn and experience. Since I came from a rural area, there was a great deal to learn. Driving was a new experience. Shopping was a new experience and having hundreds of people around all the time was a new experience. I soon learned to navigate the new environment and start work.

I was given a week to get orientated. It was good that I had some experience in the intensive care environment, but this fifteen-bed unit was a whole new ballgame. The unit received open heart patients, trauma patients, and general surgery patients. On occasion, some pediatric patients were sent to this unit because they required a high level of monitoring and care.

A nursing shortage was going on during this time. There were not enough registered nurses for each shift. So many times, each nurse had three or four critically ill patients. Sometimes, many more.

MARY LU GERKE PH.D.

Walking through the Storm

On a Saturday AM shift, I came to work to a full ICU. As shifts turned over, we always met in the conference room in the back of the unit. Two of us sat at the table, waiting for the rest of the staff to come in for the shift. Soon a technician came in. But after waiting fifteen minutes, I decided to check out what was going on. The day shift charge nurse came back to the conference room. She said that the unit was full, busy, and that there were only three of us to care for all of them. We sat there somewhat in shock. How were we going to get through the shift? More importantly, how would the patients get through the shift? I was in charge since there wasn't anyone else. I called the supervisor for help. She said she could send a nursing assistant from obstetrics. That wasn't ideal, but at this point any help was better than none.

I asked, "Can we call the head nurse?"

The supervisor said, "It's her day off. We don't call in head nurses. They are not part of the union."

I hadn't worked in a unionized facility before. I did not know that the administration from the head nurse up was not in the union. I also thought that it shouldn't make a difference if managers and head nurses were or were not part of a union; they should care about the patients and their staff enough to help.

If I would have had time, I would have run to the chapel to ask God for help. But I just raised my eyes to the sky and prayed, "Oh God, help us during this day to care for your flock."

We assigned the patients. One nurse had five patients. I took the other ten patients with the nursing assistant from obstetrics. No breaks today, I thought. Let's do this. I checked on each patient and gave the nursing assistant her duties. She could give baths and oral hygiene, basic care. The morning was insane. Physicians made rounds and expected a nurse to accompany them. Well since there was only two of us, it was a bit difficult. The physicians were not very happy. I said that if they would like to help, that would be great. They smiled and walked away.

The day continued. Just keeping up with the medication and infusions was keeping us crazy busy. Then about 1 PM, the heart monitor in room 14 alarmed. I ran to the bed to discover the patient was in ventricular fibrillation. I yelled for help and started compressions and breathing for the patient.

I yelled, "Call a code."

A code blue was announced over the PA system. Soon the physicians and nurse supervisor came. We continued with CPR, but the physician said the patient wasn't getting oxygen and he wanted to perform a tracheotomy. I ran to get the procedure tray. In the middle of the chaos, the other patients' alarms were going off and I had to direct the nursing assistant and other RN to check on all of them. I asked the nurse supervisor if she could assist with the tracheotomy, but she said she wasn't comfortable doing that. So, I assisted and we got an airway in and stabilized the heart rhythm. The patient survived and we were all very happy.

After cleaning up the room, I went back to checking in on every patient.

The day shift was over, and the PM shift had come on. They had a couple more RN staff. Their shift would be a bit better. I continued to work. Finishing all the charting and then I went to finish a couple of baths.

The PM charge nurse came over to me and said, "Why are you still here? Your shift is over."

I said, "Each one of these patients deserve to have a bath and oral care, I am going to assure that all patients are comfortable before I leave."

I left at 6P M.

As I was leaving, the PM charge nurse said to me, "You will learn that some days you have to do the minimal for the patients."

I said, "Well as long as I am able to walk, I will do the best I can for each patient."

There were many shifts like that, some worse, some better. But I learned to depend on the team. To help each patient to the best of my ability.

Wounded Healer

A day shift started routinely; the intensive care unit was almost full. The emergency room called and said they were bringing a forty-five-year-old male who had experienced a cardiac arrest at his workplace. He had been resuscitated but even though there was a heartbeat, he was not breathing on his own and was not responsive. I was assigned to this gentleman. His wife, a twelve-year-old daughter and eight-year-old son accompanied him. After we transferred him into bed, I allowed the family to come in. We took him for a scan of his brain and had an EEG done to see if he had any brain activity. Sad to say that even with the resuscitation at the scene, it was too late to save his brain.

We brought the family to the patient's bedside. The physician then came in to tell them that their husband and father had died. We would remove life support as soon as they said their good-bye. The wife sobbed and cried.

Then the little boy went over to his dad and screamed, "Dad don't leave us. We need you, Dad. I love you. You need to keep teaching me how to throw the ball and go fishing with me. Don't go, don't go."

The wife and daughter tried to console him without much luck.

I said, "I will leave you alone with your husband and dad for a while." Then I went to the stock room across from the room and cried.

The head nurse came in and said, "What are you doing?"

I looked at her with tears running down my face and said, "We just lost a patient, they just lost a husband and dad. He was only forty-five. It just doesn't seem fair."

She said, "You are a nurse. You shouldn't be so upset. We don't show our emotions like that." She walked out of the storeroom.

I shook my head and thought, if I ever am a head nurse, I will not behave like that. I will comfort the patients, families, and my staff. Compassion and empathy are part of our profession. We don't just perform tasks; we are in a special relationship with the people we serve. Healthcare providers often disregard the wounds and pain they absorb when a patient dies or when things occur that they cannot explain. There is need to heal those wounds by being still and listening to the Healer of all Healers, God.

There were many good times in the city. I made wonderful friends and experiences that would last a lifetime. But all things end, and I received information from my family that caused me to decide to move back home. I was the youngest of twelve and although I was just in my twenties, my parents were in their seventies.

When I was born, my dad said to my mom. "I'm glad we had a girl; she will take care of us in our old age."

I never forgot that story and knew that I needed to keep that promise.

There were many jobs available back home. When I called the hospital, they said I could work as a nurse educator in the ICU. The same unit I had been a staff nurse in when I left. I thought why not give it a try? Education wasn't necessarily what I had a passion for but sometimes it is good to try different roles. Nursing has many different paths to take. The vice president of nursing was a Franciscan nun and she thought this was the role I should take because I had a bachelor's degree in nursing. I would have liked the head nurse role better, but I decided to accept the nurse educator role and see what happened.

Packing up wasn't too difficult. My friend and I had only been in the "Big City" for two years and hadn't accumulated much.

On the day we were supposed to move, the moving company never showed up. I called home, frantic. Mom called my brothers and the next day, my two brothers showed up with a truck to take our belongings and us home. That's what family does. I was so thankful.

Chapter Four
Next Step Nurse Educator

I started my new job after a short break to take my parents on a vacation. It was a great time to catch up with my parents on all they had done in the past few years. I decided to live at home for a while. I needed to think through the next steps.

The nurse educator leaving orientated me to my role. Most of the work was to educate new nurses in the intensive care unit. There were classes to teach on monitoring and equipment, policies and procedures and basics of nursing care in the intensive care unit. The turnover was pretty consistent, and it seemed I was starting a new orientation every month. It was good to see all my old colleagues and I felt comfortable in the intensive care area. All the experiences from my past few years paid off. I could bring to the classes, real life experiences and examples to teach the new staff.

Educating is a critical nursing role. If staff are educated in their role, the patients are cared for safely and with compassion. The nurse educator before me never worked the night shift to orientate new staff. I didn't agree with that approach, so my orientation of staff included a week of the PM shift and a week of the night shift. There are special events that happen on each shift, and I wanted to make sure that the nurses I educated knew about them.

The other reason was to be able to practice nursing myself. During the PM and night shifts, there weren't as many nurses as possible available, and there was an opportunity to do patient care.

Many of the new nurses had not experienced taking care of a cardiac arrest patient. There wasn't always an opportunity to allow them that experience but when there was an arrest, I wanted them to be able to experience the intensity of that moment. I would ask the experienced nurses to allow the new nurse to perform tasks like defibrillation and critical medication delivery. Most of the staff were understanding and supportive.

Because I taught cardiac monitoring, I was also asked to teach in small rural clinics and hospitals. Little did I know at that time that there would be times in my future that I would revisit those same clinics and hospitals. I enjoyed meeting with the staff from those areas. The staff of those facilities wear many hats. There are no other disciplines like respiratory therapist or infusion therapy therapists. Cardiac monitoring was an expectation for the RN of those facilities as they were the first line of care for patients experiencing cardiac conditions. The other aspect of these facilities is how very grateful and appreciative they were to have someone come to teach them basic cardiac monitoring and care.

I never liked repetition. So, after I had updated all the

orientation manuals and had taught about twenty new staff, I was getting restless to pursue my dream job as a head nurse. I belonged to the local Critical Care Nursing Association and developed friendships with critical care nurses from the larger Lutheran hospital across town. During one of the meetings of the local chapter, the administrative director of the intensive care areas came and sat down by me. As the evening went along, we got to know each other better. She asked if I ever thought about working at her hospital. I said I would be open to the opportunity if the right position ever became available. She asked what position that would be.

I said, "Well my dream is to be a head nurse of an intensive care unit."

She said, "Well, you never know," and smiled.

It wasn't too many weeks later, I received a call from the administrative director asking if I would be interested in applying for the head nurse job in the intensive care unit at the Lutheran hospital. My heart jumped for joy. I said I would love to.

So, I filled out the application and went for my interview. I met with the administrative director, some staff, and the vice president of nursing. I wasn't too impressed with the vice president of nursing. When I went into his office, he had his feet up on his desk and was smoking a pipe. He asked several questions.

Finally, he asked me, "Why should I hire you as the head nurse?"

I looked him straight in the eyes and said, "I'm the best person for this job and if given the opportunity, you will see why."

The acceptance of the job was another story. I told my mom I was offered the head nurse job at the Lutheran Hospital.

She said, "You're not going to accept it, are you?"

I said, "I think I would like to."

She said, "But you're Catholic and should serve the Catholic institutions."

I was taken aback by her position, but I really wanted this job.

The administrative director called to ask if I had decided. I said almost.

She said, "Let me take you out for dinner and we can discuss your concerns and help you decide."

She took me to a very beautiful restaurant. A few other people were a long at the dinner that I knew from the Critical Care Nursing chapter. After listening to them and how very desperate they were for new leadership, I decided to take the job. I just hoped that God would understand. I knew he loved all people and wanted us to serve all his sheep. I listened deeply to my inner self and knew this was my path.

Before I left the Catholic hospital, the vice president

of nursing asked me to come to lunch. I wasn't expecting lunch to be served on a fine linen covered table in a private conference room. Sister Joyce was a wonderful mentor to me, and it was hard to leave her flock. We had a great conversation. She told me that she had actually worked at the Lutheran hospital across town before she went into the convent.

When I told her my mom wasn't happy that I was going to work there, she said, "There are great people who work there, and you will be just fine. If you ever want to come back here, we would love to have you."

Then I knew for sure that the decision was the right one. I would use her guidance in the future when things got tough.

Now, I needed to prepare for a new hospital, a new role, and new staff. I pulled together some of my diaries from when I started the nursing path. I just let them speak to me and how I should approach this new step. I read about the great mentors, head nurses, and colleagues who inspired me along the way. I also read about head nurses and colleagues who I would not want to replicate.

Then I was inspired by an article, "The Way of the Shepherd" by Leman and Pentak (2004). This would be my foundation as a head nurse in the intensive care unit.

Chapter Five

Walking and Living the Dream

Leading Nurses Like a Shepherd

The morning of my first day as head nurse, I dressed in a scrub top and pants and in my white nursing shoes. I was greeted in the conference room by the interim head nurse and the staff from the shift. I was going to be oriented to the intensive care unit. It was a fifteen-bed unit. The morning I started, the unit was full of patients and very busy. The interim head nurse seemed to less than welcoming and I needed to find out why. What I discovered was that she, along with the night charge nurse, had applied for the position. They, of course, were disappointed. I knew I would need to gain their trust. At first, I just listened to it and became comfortable in the space. The intensive care unit in the metropolitan city gave me a great background for the patients in this unit.

The unit was so busy and the person who was orientated me was called back to give patient care and relieve nurses for a break. I said I would be fine, and this gave me time to explore on my own. I went into the dirty utility room. At that time, all bed basins, bed pans, and emesis basins were cleaned and sterilized in the dirty utility room. I went into the room. The basins and pans were stacked to the ceiling. I thought this was very bad. I started washing the basins and pans. Soon, I had most of them cleaned and ready to be sterilized.

The nurse orientating me came in the room and said, "What are you doing?"

I said, "Cleaning the equipment."

She said, "Nurses don't do that."

I smiled and said, "I just thought I would help. I know how to wash and clean equipment."

We then headed out for the rest of the day.

Orientation was brief but I was given an office space with all the manuals, policies, and scheduling materials. I had never did scheduling of a whole staff. I sought out other head nurses in the hospital who were more than willing to help.

Getting to know the new unit, new staff and new role would take some time but I was willing to go through the process.

I met with the fifty staff members individually. I asked them three questions.

What is your background?

What are your goals and dreams?

What do you expect of me as your head nurse?

The process took a few weeks to complete. I spent time on the PM shift and then the night shift.

My session with the two candidates who had interviewed for the head nurse position was both different and insightful. Both nurses were very clear that they did not respect the previous head nurse. I asked why. They said she was never available to help and that she was very close friends with the administrative director and vice president of nursing.

The unit was very short staffed, and the turnover rate was greater than fifty percent a year. There were not enough expert staff and many novice staff. The nurses and support staff seemed overwhelmed and anxious causing confusion, frustration, and compassion fatigue. Although there were many factors that nurses leave their department and facilities, the major factor is the leader.

I read and learned that understanding complexity and chaos concepts is one way to decrease anxiety and increase focus. Increased technology, ever changing knowledge, and change causes the illusion that we are out of control. There needs to be simplicity brought to the minds of the nurses in the midst of complexity and chaos. How do I help the staff to regain focus and core nursing values? Nurses need to build not only technical skills but also the capacity to develop their minds, emotions, and spirits of caring for the patients.

Seasoned nurses must grab the opportunity to transfer knowledge and wisdom about developing skills and relationships with the patients and families to novice nurses. Most importantly, to learn the art of being fully present with each patient and family.

I turned to the article called, "The Way of the Shepherd"

by Leman and Pertak (2004) to put into action leadership skills that were needed to change the intensive Ccre unit. I also reflected on Psalm 23 of the Catholic Bible, "The Lord is my Shepherd". These materials inspired me to lead the nursing staff like a shepherd leads the flock.

There are seven ancient secrets shared in the book that I applied not only to leadership but to caring for and serving our patients. Exploring these <u>seven principles</u> lights the way to focusing on the important core values of caring, nursing and leadership. I set out to use these principles as guideposts in my practice as a leader.

Know the Condition of Your Flock

Nursing leaders now more than ever need to know every nurse that they are responsible for leading. There are many tools, methods, forms that help with performance appraisal, mentoring, and precepting of staff. But it is not just completing the list, it is the process of eliciting this information that makes the difference. The staff needs to feel and know that the nursing leaders are completely present for them and not distracted by the "to do" lists we are obsessed by and held accountable for. I listened to chief nursing officers in the country saying that the financial bottom lines and chief financial officers were driving the bus. Therefore, it is even more important now to find fully present moments with our nurses. Not just for them but for us. They need to know that being present for each and every one of them is a priority. So, when you meet with staff, shut off the cell phone, computer, and pressing agendas to fully be with them in their world. Better than that go to where they work. They need to experience the presence of the nurse leader. I decided I needed to work side by side with them at the moment. Then I would be able to:

Learn about the nurses, one nurse at a time.

Develop a priority plan that is driven by the staff and the patients.

Engage the nurses on a regular basis by rounding and staff meetings.

Work side by side with the staff, doing patient care to role model.

Keep your eyes and ears open, question, and follow through on promises.

These elements call for nurse leaders to be fully present with the staff as we expect them to be fully present with the patient – one at a time, one moment at a time.

Discover the Shape of Your Sheep

The shepherd leader needs to develop the SHAPE of the staff by applying an individualized approach to each nurse. This simple approach assures each nurse sees the nurse leader as a mentor to assessment and individualized presence. I used SHAPE from "The Way of the Shepherd" by Leman and Pentak (2004). Then applied nursing concepts and principles to the concept.

S – Strengths – What does each nurse bring to the unit? Are you assessing the strengths to place the individual in the environment that will have the best opportunity to succeed? Are their views and priorities aligned with my vision, organizational mission, and strategies? If not, I needed to have a dialogue with the staff person to discover why or why not. Sometimes the staff (sheep) are in the wrong pasture.

H – Heart – What is each nurse passionate about? Is this passion being utilized to its full extent? Have you shared your passion with the staff? How often?

A - Attitude – Leaders want and need people with good attitudes. Leman and Pentak (2004) share that people with positive attitudes make better team players. In fact, when given a choice between talent and a positive attitude, choosing a positive attitude brings the best return on investment.

Do I promote a positive attitude and energy when I am present with the staff? Jean Watson, a national nursing leader contends that the energy we emit in the patient's room affects the attitude and energy of the patient. The same principle can be applied to our staff. Positive energy and attitude are contagious. Focusing on healing and understanding is a method to promote engaged and positive staff.

P – Personality – Each nurse is different, each has their own stories, own history, and own values. Do we recognize that and seek to discover how to accept the difference as a good thing and use the unique individual talents to enrich our units, departments, and organization? Experts on inclusion and diversity conclude that recognizing the uniqueness and need for a variety of perspectives brings a richer and more complete plan and outcome.

E – Experiences - Often key to understanding nurses is the stories of what they experience. I started storytelling at most of our meetings and our organizational nursing staff meetings. Stories are shared, some of success and some stories of less than positive outcomes. Both types teach the staff how the experience brought learning and enrichment to the parties involved. I encouraged them to take time to understand the perspective and stories. It would teach and also fulfill them. The bottom line of shape was:

Your choice of nurses can make managing and leading the unit, department, organization easier or harder.

Know the SHAPE of your nurses – make sure they are in the right unit, department, organization, and position.

Help Your Sheep Identify with You

Developing relationships can be easy for some and difficult

for others. But relationship building with our colleagues and staff is what leadership is all about. Do my nurses know who I am? Do they know my vision, my values as a professional nurse, my dreams, and aspirations? Nurses need to know their leaders well and become their colleague in pursuit of the values, mission and outcome of the unit, department, and organization.

So, I decided to apply the following:

Build trust with the nurses – one at a time.

Model authenticity, integrity, and compassion.

Set high standards of performance.

Relentlessly communicate my values and sense of mission.

Define the cause of each individual and tell them how they affect the values and mission.

Leadership isn't just professional, it's personal.

Make Your Pasture a Safe Place

No other time in history has safety in health care had so much focus and concern. Our environment does not only mean the physical layout, although that is important. Safety includes the processes, procedures, and policies we put into place to keep the patient and environment safe. Because we are in the information world – never out of touch – we have ready resources to review best practices, adaptive and innovative processes, procedures, and policies. When the standards are in place the hard part comes. We must hold each other accountable to follow them. It is not only the manager's responsibility; it is every nurse and team member who works on the unit or organization.

The principles below help ensure that safety is kept in the forefront.

Keep your staff well informed.

Infuse every position with importance.

Stay focused on the mission – do not get distracted.

Deal with colleagues and individuals who are instigators or don't fulfill the mission.

Consider rotating nurses through a variety of experiences and positions.

Stay visible.

Don't give problems time to fester - follow through on issues as soon as possible.

The Staff of Direction - Responsibility to Direct People

After reading the book, *The Way of the Shepherd* (Leman & Pentake, 2004), I researched the shepherd's rod and staff, it is like a walking stick. My investigation led me to buy a traditional shepherd's staff to remind me of my role and the importance of nursing leadership. The shepherd's staff has a curved end which is called the hook and used to pull or guide the individual sheep to go the right direction. It is a gentle nudge or pull around the sheep's neck to get them to go the right direction. Often sheep focus on the here and now – the green grass, and they don't realize the pasture or what's further in front of them. That is a great analogy of what nursing leaders must do. Sometimes, nurses are so absorbed in the day-to-day work they are unable to see the vision and goals of the unit or organization. There need to be frequent, gentle nudges and pulls to help them stay together and on a safe, caring path. This consistent vigilance delivers staff who trust the nursing leader. The shepherd or nursing leader in this case is responsible for keeping an eye on the horizon. Nursing staff put their wellbeing into our hands. They look to us for guidance on decision making, problem solving, and mentoring. We need to offer education; options and guidance that help nurses make professional patient care decisions as well as personal professional decisions. Through knowing each nurse as described before, we can share our experiences and wisdom to guide them in making wise choices. We are the conduit between all the disciplines, medicine, administration, and the nursing staff. Help colleagues critically think through an issue and prioritize the work. If an individual nurse is exhibiting problems deal with them until resolved.

Know where your staff is going – stay in front of the changes, best practices and adaptive models

that lead the staff to a caring and safe environment.

When directing or questioning, use persuasion, not coercion.

Give your nurses choices and freedom to be an active partner in developing standards, policies, and professional models of care.

Help your interdisciplinary team to be relentless in delivery high quality, safe care 100% of the time.

Remind yourself and others that failure is not fatal – just lessons learned.

The Rod of Correction – Responsibility to Correct People

When gentle nudging and encouragement doesn't seem to work, a firmer, more directive approach is required. Instead of the hook, shepherds use the straight end of the shepherd's staff or a rod. Probably, one of the most difficult and often misused tools in leadership is discipline and threatening behavior toward staff. However, a firm approach is not a soft method; it sends the message that counseling, disciplinary action or termination in some cases is the best for the individual as well as the staff or organization. It isn't an easy job. The rod or discipline can be underused or overused. If used too often, staff are driven by fear and mistrust. Used too infrequently, the staff runs every which way without direction. Remember each nurse is an individual and thus responds to various leadership methods. Some staff need a firmer, clearer directive. Other nurses respond better to the hook and guidance. However, in both methods there is a need to always take the opportunity to teach and learn from each situation.

Protect – stand in the gap and fight for the nurses.

Correct – approach discipline as a teaching and learning opportunity.

Inspect – regularly seek out information from nurses and the team about their progress.

The staff needed to know there are red lines that cannot be breached. I shared my red lines:

All patients, families, and colleagues are to be respected.

Listen, listen, listen! Don't spontaneously respond.

Think before you act.

The nurse is a patient and family advocate.

Patient perspective is the most important.

Follow physician orders. Question the physician to understand.

The patient and families come first before our own needs.

There were sometimes when I needed to terminate a nurse. These were very difficult. I had a friend who told me. "If firing an employee is easy for you, it's time for you to leave the position."

One example of terminating an employee was during a busy shift. It was so busy I was working as a staff nurse and caring for patients. I was in a patient's room which was separated from the next patient only by a curtain. One of my staff nurses was taking care of the patient next to me. I heard yelling and screaming coming from that room. I went over to investigate. The nurse was swearing at the patient. Using foul language. I was shocked. Family members were present. I needed to intervene. I asked the nurse if I could see her in my office. I went and got someone to watch our patients and apologized to the patient and family. Then I went to my office. The nurse was sitting waiting for me.

I closed the door. I said, "What was that all about?"

She said, "The patient was upset and not following my directions."

"Many of our patients get upset," I said. "You are a professional nurse and when patients and families get upset, they need compassionate, caring nurses."

She just sat there with a bit of a smirk on her face. No tears, no regrets.

I asked, "Do you have anything else you would like to say?"

"Not really," she said.

I paused for a moment. "OK, then you can clean out

your locker and report to the human resources department down the hall. I will call them and let them know you are coming."

She gasped, "Surely you're kidding."

"No Beth, I'm not kidding," I said. "I am really sorry, but our patients and families come first, and you crossed a red line. Disrespect will not be tolerated in this unit."

She said, "We already are short of staff. Who will take care of my patients today?"

I looked her straight in the eyes and said, "I will."

After Beth left, I took a moment and just cried. It was the first time I had to fire a nurse, but sadly, it would not be the last. I thought about my role and I knew I had to keep the patients, family, and staff safe and respected.

The Heart of the Shepherd

Nursing is a privileged profession. People who are called to this profession must carry with them compassion, passion, and persistence. The heart of nursing is staying focused on the patient and family. When we tack on leadership, we should not let that focus be lost. We need to lead by example with passion and compassion. We need to set aside the distractions of our busy agendas to see nurses one at a time – being fully present. When meeting with each other, we need to take a deep breath and focus with full attention to the individual in our presence.

Walking in the Shoes of the Patient and Family

After I had been head nurse for about a year, I was in early morning report. One of the nurses came into the conference room and said she needed to talk to me. I stepped out into the hallway with her.

She looked at me and said, "I have some bad news, your dad collapsed in the barn at the farm. The ambulance was called and they are taking him to the hospital."

I knew they would take him to the Catholic hospital, so I ran to my car to meet them in the emergency room. When I got there, they had taken him to one of the rooms. Mom, my sister, and brother were with him. I came in and walked up to dad's bedside.

He looked at me with his big blue eyes. He said, "It's bad, isn't it?'

"I don't know Dad," I said.

He said, "I know it's bad; we have talked about this. You know what to do if I can't walk down to the barn again."

I gave him a big hug. Tears ran down my cheeks and I wiped tears from his cheeks. "You're in a great place dad. They will do everything possible," I said.

The Catholic hospital did not have a CT scanner, so Dad had to be taken across town to the Lutheran hospital where I worked. I told Mom to wait there, and I would go over to the hospital and meet Dad in the CT scan room.

When Dad arrived, he had been intubated to help his breathing. That was a surprise to me. They said he was deteriorating quickly. I stood outside the CT scanner as they positioned him for the scan. One person came up to me and put his arm around me. I turned to see a radiologist I had worked with for many years.

He said, "I'll stay here with you as we do the head scan."

The machine buzzed and soon an image of Dad's brain started appearing. I couldn't believe it. The radiologist looked at me.

He said, "You have seen this before, but it wasn't your dad. There is a life-ending intracerebral bleed." He continued, "You know that there isn't any intervention we can do but to keep him comfortable."

Dad was unconscious and would no longer be able to communicate. They took Dad back to the Catholic hospital. I drove back to meet Mom and my family in the intensive care unit waiting room. I had been with families when they received bad news many times. But this was different; this was my family. I went into the waiting room. All of my siblings were there except one. I went over to my mom. I hugged her as we both cried.

"Isn't there anything we can do?" she asked.

I said, "No Mom, all we can do is pray."

My one sister, who wasn't there was a Catholic nun in Superior, Wi. We arranged to fly home and my two brothers-in-law picked her up at the airport. During the next few hours, our family of twelve stood around my dad's bed. The doctors wanted to know if we wanted to put dad on a breathing machine to keep him alive until my sister arrived. Mom didn't think Dad would have wanted that. Soon, he was breathing shallowly and then his heart slowed and stopped. When my sister came, Dad had died but was still in the intensive care unit. She was the second oldest. She went over to Dad, held his hand, and cried. The pain of losing a father is numbing. I guess I never even thought he was going to die. All of the pain and sorrow I put in my heart to remember when I cared for patients and families going through the death journey.

Comforting the Dying

As a nurse leader, there are many ways to teach. One way is by example. One day, we were notified by the emergency room that there had been a motor vehicle accident. An elderly woman and her husband were involved in the accident. The woman did not survive the accident, but the husband had minor injuries. They were bringing the woman's body to ICU so the family could view and say their last goodbyes.

I instructed them to bring the body to our procedure room. Then I asked a staff nurse to get me a basin of warm water, soap, towels, and warm blankets.

The staff nurse looked at me like I had lost my mind and said, "Why? She's dead."

I replied, "Yes, she is dead, but her husband of thirty-five years is coming to see his wife for the last time. When he touches her, I want him to touch a warm hand and face."

They brought the body. The woman (wife) had many cuts, bruises, and bloody abrasions. The staff nurse and I washed and dressed the wounds as best we could. Then we covered the body with many warm blankets.

I told the husband and family they could come to view their wife and mother. Since the husband was elderly, they brought him in a wheelchair. They wheeled him next to the gurney that held his wife. The first thing the husband did was reach for his wife's hand.

Tears ran down his cheeks and he looked at me and said, "Oh my goodness, she is still warm." He stood up, kissed his wife, and said, "Rest now in the palm of God's hands."

After the family had time with their wife and mother, I sat down with the staff nurse.

"Now do you understand why it was important to wash and warm the body?" I asked.

"Yes," the staff nurse said, "I will never forget this incident. Thanks."

Special moments for patients and families are also special moments for the nurses and healthcare workers.

But to receive those gifts, we need to be open to creating these relationships. When anyone loses a loved one, we must think and feel how we would be in that situation. Sometimes nurses need to put an arm around the person grieving and cry with them. Sometimes saying a prayer together will help. Sometimes just being with them in silence shows respect and support. We need to use our inner spirit and intuition to know what will help those left behind.

Listening to Messages from Angels

It was a cold, snowy December day. The intensive care unit was busy. We received a call from the emergency room, they were bringing a seventy-year-old male who had a skiing accident. I prepared the room and waited for the patient. When they brought the patient, he was not breathing on his own. The emergency room nurse was using a breathing bag as they transferred him. We connected the patient to a ventilator. The patient's name was Joe. He was a minister at one of our local churches.

His son explained to me what had happened. He said, "The snow was so beautiful, light, and fluffy. My dad loves to ski. He was skiing down one of the most difficult slopes; I was right behind him when he fell. I rushed to see if he was OK. When I got to his side, he was not breathing. I started doing mouth to mouth resuscitation. Thank God there were ski patrols in the area.

They brought a gurney, and we brought him down the slope to the ski lodge. The ambulance came and now we are here."

The CT scan revealed that Joe had severed his spinal cord right below the back of his head. These injuries are life-threatening. The spinal cord could no longer communicate from the head to the rest of the body, including the breathing. The doctor explained the situation to the son and wife. Since Joe was unresponsive when he was admitted, there was a chance he may never regain consciousness. The son and wife stood at Joe's side, stunned and crying. It would take a few days to see if there were any indications that Joe would regain consciousness but regardless, Joe would never have any function of his body from the neck down.

I wondered what I could do as Joe's nurse to ease the son and wife's grief. So, for some reason, I think it was my guardian angel who put the words in my mouth. As I cared for Joe, I just started asking about Joe, the man.

"So, tell me about your dad and husband," I asked.

The son said, "He was a minister; he helped so many people. My dad loved the outdoors and being active. He loved piano music and often asked me to play for him."

"My son is a concert pianist," the wife said.

I continued the conversations with them and developed a clear picture of who Joe was.

On the third day, Joe seemed to be responding and

eventually he opened his eyes. There was so much happiness for his son and wife. But the doctor would sooner or later need to tell Joe that he would never move on his own again. After Joe started becoming more aware of what had happened and where he was, we taught him to indicate yes and no answers by blinking his eyes once for yes and twice for no.

The doctor thought it was time to tell Joe the prognosis. The doctor also had the bioethicist present. He wanted to assure everyone, including himself, that the patient was able to understand and comprehend the prognosis message.

Joe's wife held his hand on one side of the bed. His son held his hand on the other side of the bed.

The doctor said, "Joe you had a ski accident. When you fell skiing, you injured your neck. Joe, you severed your spinal cord at the level of your third vertebrae."

Joe stared at the doctor.

The doctor continued, "What that means, Joe, is that you are paralyzed from your neck down. You will not be able to breath on your own; you will not be able to talk, you will not be able to feed yourself or move any of your limbs."

The doctor asked Joe to indicate yes if he understood. All of us watched.

A tear ran down Joe's face. He blinked his eyes once, indicating he understood.

Everyone left and the wife and son stayed with Joe. It was a lot to comprehend, and we thought it best for them to just be alone together for a while.

The bioethicist and doctor discussed the next steps. Joe and his family would need to decide to continue keeping Joe alive or to stop further intervention. There are many cases where the patient decides to stay on a ventilator and tube feedings. There are other cases where the patient decides to be taken off life support.

We talked to the wife and son in the conference room. We explained the options. We could keep Joe on a ventilator, tube feeding, and all the equipment to support him. He would be taken to a rehabilitation center or nursing home. The other option the patient and family had was to remove all life support and keep Joe comfortable until he died.

Joe's wife and son both agreed that Joe would not want to live if he were dependent on equipment with no hope for recovery. They decided to present the options to Joe. The bioethicist, doctor, and nurse returned to Joe's room to deliver the options. After explaining the options to Joe, they asked Joe which option he wanted. Option one, to continue to support him with equipment. Joe blinked twice indicating no. Option two, to discontinue life support. Joe blinked once indicating yes. To determine that Joe was of sound mind, the bioethicist performed a series of tests to assure Joe was of sound mind.

We spent time with the wife and son to determine how they would spend the last days and hours with their loving husband and father.

The wife said, "Could we get a piano here, so Joe's son could play for him?"

I told them to bring pictures that meant the most to Joe. We hung them everywhere around the room. Now to get a piano. I decided we could bring the piano up from the lobby.

The tech that worked with me said, "How and who would give us permission to do that?"

I said, "Hmm, I don't think we have time to get permission from administration. We are going to bring it up this evening after everyone is gone."

The tech smiled. "OK, I'm in."

The PM shift came on and I stayed with Joe and his family.

Then I said to the tech, "Let's go get the piano."

He smiled and accompanied me to the lobby. Although it was a bit difficult, we got the piano on the large elevator and brought the piano into Joe's room. This was the first time I saw Joe smile.

The wife, in tears, said, "Thank you so much."

The son sat down by the piano and started to play. It was beautiful. I notified the doctor bioethicist and anesthesiologist that Joe and the family were ready to discontinue the life support systems. With wonderful music filling the room, we started to discontinue the monitor, intravenous tubes, and other equipment. Then the anesthesiologist gave Joe a minor sedative to ease his anxiety. Finally, we discontinued the ventilator. The room was filled with an aura of peace and love. I felt the glow of light and peaceful silence. I looked out the window and saw large snowflakes falling. Like angel feathers. I knew Joe was at peace.

Captain of the Ship

I loved being the head nurse of the intensive care unit. But there were times when I didn't think I would be able to make it through another day. The unit was short staffed. I remembered that Saturday in the metropolitan hospital when the head nurse didn't come in to help us. There were many times I would work sixteen and even twenty-four hours with the staff, caring for patients. One time, I had stayed and cared for patients on the day shift and PM shift. I left the unit around 11:30 PM. The shower felt great, and I climbed into bed. The phone rang around 1:30 AM. I always answered the phone in case it was the intensive care unit.

"Hello," I said.

"Hi, this Joe, the night charge nurse. We have a situation here, and I would like you to come in," he said.

"What's going on?" I asked.

"Dr. B screamed and yelled at one of the families of

the patient who has been determined brain dead. You know the one who was in the motor vehicle accident."

"I'll be right in," I said.

So much for a good night's sleep. I put my scrub uniform on and headed back to the hospital.

When I arrived, and was entering the intensive care unit, I was greeted by Dr. B.

"We need to talk," he said.

"Indeed, we do," I said.

He went on to explain that the patient had been brain dead for three days and that we were keeping him alive with equipment and fluids. He felt that it was a waste of time and energy.

"When I left last evening," I said, "the family said they were waiting until his sister arrived from California."

"That is just crazy," Dr. B said. "He isn't going to respond to her anyway. So, what's the difference if he is dead or alive?"

I couldn't believe what I was hearing.

Dr. B. continued, "You know in Argentina, where I practiced, the doctor was the captain of the shift. When we gave orders, they were followed, no matter what."

I took him into the coffee room so others would not hear. As we walked to the coffee room, I thought how I should respond to him. Then out of nowhere it came to me.

"Listen Dr. B.," I said. "First of all, you are not in Argentina, you are in United States. And you might be the captain of the ship, but the patient and family own the ship. They are why we are here, and they are paying our salaries. So, this is what we are going to do; you and I are going to meet with the family in the conference room. You will apologize to them and then we will find out when they believe his sister will arrive."

He didn't say another word. To this day, I believe God was speaking through me. We met with the family, and they appreciated the apology. The sister would be arriving in the morning and then we would proceed to remove the life support.

After a few years in the head nurse role, I was eager to continue my own education. A colleague suggested I attend the master's degree program with her only thirty minutes away from home. I applied for the program and started another step on the nursing path. The degree was a master's in nursing administration. I was able to attend part time and work full time. I attended evening classes for five years. During this time, the vice president of nursing at my hospital was a great support and mentor. Sometimes I didn't think I could make it. But I now had a strong nursing staff and great supportive colleagues. The completion of my master's degree was another milestone along my path in nursing and leadership.

Chapter Six

If Not You, Who?

Our deepest fear is not that we are inadequate.

Our deepest fear is that we are powerful beyond measure.

It is our light, not our darkness, that most frightens us.

We ask ourselves, "Who am I to be brilliant, gorgeous, talented, and fabulous?"

Actually, who are you not to be?

Your playing small does not serve the world.

Marianne Williamson

The vice-president of nursing called me into her office. This vice president was new to the position, but I knew her as a colleague for many years. I finished up my work in the intensive care unit and walked to her office.

She welcomed me and she said, "I asked you here to help me resolve a major issue."

That piqued my interest and I waited to hear how I could help.

She continued, "You're aware that our administrative director of the operating room area has left. There are over 150 employees in that area. The pre-operative and recovery areas along with the anesthesia department is also included under what the administrative director covered." The vice president continued, "I was wondering if you would be willing to take over that area as an interim assignment."

I asked, "What about the intensive care unit?"

"You would still be leading that area too," she said.

"Wow," I said. "That is over 300 employees I would have report to me."

She smiled and said, "If not you, who?"

That sealed the deal. I knew it would be a very difficult job. I also knew I had the skills and knowledge to do it.

Patient and Families come First!

I became a member of nursing organizations and attended many nursing conferences and workshops. On one occasion while I was attending a conference, I was called to the front desk for a phone call. My heartbeat fast; I thought something had happened to my family. I picked up the phone.

The person calling was the physician who was head of the aesthesia department. He was very upset. He said, "What do you think you are doing by giving up your office for a family waiting room?"

I was given a nice office with windows outside of the intensive care unit. Our families did not have a waiting room close to the unit. I decided to move my office to a small area in the library. I did not need a big office more than our families needed a waiting room close to the intensive care unit.

I gave Dr. C. the explanation.

He said, "I want that space for my office. I am going to talk to the vice president.

I responded, "Go ahead, but I thought the patients and families always came first. Besides, I'm sure you know I am at a conference. Was it really that urgent?"

I knew this would not be the end of it. Not too long after I got a call from the vice president. She said Dr. C had been to her office and was very angry about the office – waiting room situation. I explained why I had done what I had done.

She said, "When you get back, perhaps we should sit down with him."

I agreed.

When I returned, I met with the vice president and Dr. C. I had decided not to back down. I said our patients' families needed a private space, especially when they were dealing with critical situations and the death of a loved one. The vice president supported my position.

That night when I got home, I received a call from Dr. C. He started all over again, about how he needed that office.

I said, "We can talk more about it tomorrow." Then I hung up the phone.

The next day, I was asked to go to the vice president's office. She said Dr. C had called her and said I had hung up on him. I said I had.

She started smiling. She said, "I told him you would not back down. Then she said, "He said you didn't care about the patients." She said, "I told him that he crossed the line, that you were one of the most caring nurses and head nurse."

I sat there, very sad. No one had ever said that about me.

The vice president said, "I told him the office would be a family waiting room, and that I would find him another office space."

I left her office and went back to the intensive care unit to give patients care.

That evening, Dr. C. called again.

He said, "Don't hang up. I'm just calling to apologize. The vice president said you were upset about my comments regarding patient concern. I didn't mean that. Can we meet tomorrow and start our relationship over?"

I said of course we could meet, and I thanked him for the apology.

We actually became close over the years. We had mutual respect for each other from that experience on.

I learned the importance of listening to other perspectives but then always focusing on our values and mission relating to the patient and family always coming first.

Help me, Help you!

The operating room department I now was administrative director over was struggling with turnover of staff and low morale. I conducted nominal sessions and listening sessions to figure out all the concerns and issues the staff was facing. I wondered how to approach all the changes needed to restore a sense of ownership and peace in the department. For many days, I read and thought about how to turn negative energy into a positive, creative flow. During that time, I was watching my two-year-old great nephew learning how to make cookies. He was very curious and wanted to be in the middle of baking. He wanted to be able to make cookie dough go into balls just like his mom was able to do.

After several attempts, Ethan looked at his mom and said, "Mom, help me, help you."

Suddenly, it hit me. I needed to be a reflective beginner with the department. I needed to be vulnerable and let them teach me how to help them. I recognized that I was not an expert in their specialty and that the answer to creating an efficient, effective, and positive team was not going to be found in me, but in them. They had the answers; all I needed to do was gain their trust and have them become the owners of the department, to be both the department staff and owners of the work.

The first staff meeting I attended told me the story of how the department had gotten to a point of despair. The room was set up in a horseshoe fashion. The clinical manager sat at the front and center of the staff. No one sat near her. When I came in, I sat between two of the staff members. Both looked oddly at me. I wondered if I had food on my face from lunch.

I said, "What's the problem?"

They said, "Oh nothing, but the last administrative director never came to our staff meeting."

The clinical manager started the staff meeting by giving updates and information about changes in policy and procedures. A couple of the staff members gave reports. Then the meeting was going to end. I thought it very strange that no one asked questions or commented on what was going on in the department.

I took advantage of the captive audience and said, "You know, I'm curious about how all of you are feeling now that the union vote is done and was turned down."

One hand after another came up. Tentatively at first, the group conversation escalated. Some said they didn't want to or enjoy coming to work anymore.

I decided to share my goal with them, "Over the next several months we are going to develop an environment that would have you wanting to come to work again. And to see work as exciting and fulfilling."

After the meeting, I stopped and talked to the staff

nurses who I had sat by during the beginning of the meeting. I asked them why they had really looked at me so strangely at the beginning of the meeting.

They told me, "We expected you to sit next to the manager, not amongst the staff."

This broke my heart. To think that such a small action meant so much to this staff. It was apparent they needed to be valued, respected, and cared about.

Numerous changes occurred over the next several months. I asked the staff to help me, help them. The initial step was to find a manager who could be a cheerleader, mentor, and servant leader. The staff was part of the interviewing and screening for the new manager. After several interviews, we found an outstanding leader. She was enthusiastic and genuinely loved the operating room area. She was both a scrub nurse and circulating nurse for surgeries.

She created the following guiding principles with the staff:

Members of the department are free to ask questions of anyone.

Work can be fun.

Decisions meet individual and department needs as much as possible.

Sharing of stories is welcomed and important.

Curiosity is encouraged and rewarded.

There is no one "right way", all ideas are valued and

need to be investigated.

Patience and tolerance is the norm.

Creativity and diversity are nurtured.

The understanding of system thinking and wholeness is embraced.

Staff will lead, teach, and learn.

We all will stretch and go outside of our comfort zone.

The new head nurse held her first staff meeting. I was a bit anxious about how it would go. She entered the room and sat on the floor in the middle of the circle of staff. She shared from her heart her hopes and dreams for the operating room. She empathized with them regarding the past few years, and how difficult it must have been for all staff. At the end of the meeting, she asked if there was anything else anyone wanted to share.

One staff member raised her hand and said, "For the first time in many years, I feel good about coming to work. A long time ago we used to feel like a family. I feel like our family is coming home."

This is what a learning-reflective leader does. The leader inspires the group to be creative followers, to be expressive staff, not passive staff. To feel not just think, and to be not just do.

I continued to also be the head nurse for the intensive care unit, but it soon became apparent that I could not do that job as well as being an administrative director. Evaluating and guiding all the staff from the intensive care unit, operating room, pre-operative area, recovery area and anesthesia department was just not possible. I decided to hire a head nurse for the intensive care unit. This was really hard. I was energized by giving patient care. Giving up this part of my practice was a step that I needed to take but would really miss. I still made rounds on patients but was not able to give total patient care that I had given over for over thirty years.

Mom – The Promise

Dad passed eighteen years ago, but I always remember the promise he made to Mom when I was born: "This little girl will care for us in our old age."

My mom missed Dad every day since he passed. Although she continued to love and care for her family, she just wasn't truly happy. When I moved back from the metropolitan city, I bought a house near work. I called Mom every day and visited her often. It came the time when she needed someone with her most of the time. My sister, who lived close by the farm, took care of Mom every day, helping her with her bath and meals. Our family met with Mom, and we decided the best thing would be to have someone live at home with her. My siblings looked at me as they all had heard the promise, and I was not married, so would be the best option. I sold my house and moved home. The farm was just five miles from the hospital. I worked during the day and then cared for Mom at night. My sister still came every day to care for Mom and my brother was around during the day running the farm.

During the first year, we developed a good routine and Mom was always very grateful. As time went on, Mom started to deteriorate. The nights were hard for her. I would tuck her in her bed with water at the bedside but after an hour or two, she needed to get up to go to the bathroom. We got a commode, so she didn't have to walk to the bathroom. I put a bell at her bedside so she could ring it when she needed me to help her get up. Some nights I was getting less than three hours of sleep. My days at work would always be at least ten hours.

One night, Mom was having a very bad night and as soon as I would get back to bed, she would ring the bell. I went into her room and got her up to the commode. I asked her what she needed from me. She just looked at me with her big brown eyes.

A tear ran down her cheek and she said, "I just need you to love me."

Then both of us were crying. I learned a great deal during the time I got to spend with my mom. She prayed a lot, and I could tell she was becoming closer to God. I realized that she was teaching me how to love deeply, to practice patience. I learned to practice, tolerance, and persistence. Mom taught me how to let go of material things and cling to spiritual things. I felt like a trapeze artist swinging from one side of the arena to the other. I felt in the middle of the past and the future.

Mom's back pain worsened, and her mobility decreased. She slept most of the time except when we needed to get her to the commode. She became weaker and weaker. At one point, we took her to the hospital because she was so weak. Her blood count was very low. They wanted to keep her at the hospital overnight and give her blood. My sister stayed the night with her. I went home and got to have a night without interruption.

I went back to the hospital the next morning.

Mom called me over to her. She grabbed my hand and said, "Take me home."

She did not want any more done. We arranged for hospice to come to her home. We arranged for a hospital bed to make it more comfortable for her.

We all knew Mom was experiencing her last days. Every year we had a family get-together at the homestead. This year we decided to have it, even though Mom was nearing the end. We thought it would be good for her and the family to say their goodbyes and spend some time with her. She was comfortable in her bed and was able to see out the front room window with all her family having a picnic and enjoying each other. It was a good day.

The next day, I was sitting by her side, and she said, "Do you see the bridge?"

I said, "What bridge?"

She continued, "The bridge covered with hibiscus flowers, and look, there is Dad."

She fell back to sleep. I called my sister, and she came over. I knew it would not be too long. Her pain was now controlled with morphine and Ativan. We called the priest to give her the last blessings.

The next day, her doctor came to the farm. Doctors usually didn't make house calls, but he and Mom had grown close together.

He took her hand and Mom said, "You are just like a son to me. Thank you for all you have done for me over the years."

A tear ran down his face and he said, "And you are like a mother to me."

The vigil continued for the next couple of days. We made mom's handprint on a paper for all the children. My siblings came and went throughout the day. Slowly, Mom became unresponsive. The death rattle is hard to listen to, but part of the dying process. Suctioning the saliva helps for brief moments but does not totally stop the rattle.

At 3:00 AM, we turned Mom to her right side, her favorite side. My brother said we should go outside for a moment. He wanted to show us something. We went outside. It was a clear night. In the sky, the brightest star lit up the night.

He said, "I think that is Dad, calling Mom home."

At 3:45 AM, Mom went to her eternal home. Explaining the loss of a parent is hard to explain. It is so difficult. We all experience it and then we understand how it feels and how to have empathy for others.

I was able to spend another year at the homestead while we settled the estate. There were many hard days, but soon I needed to move on.

Moving on

Starting a doctoral program was a very difficult decision. I had been away from academia for three years. It was a relief to just do a full-time job and not go home to work on schoolwork. A close colleague of mine over the years had finished her PhD degree in human and organizational development and introduced me to the idea of enrolling in that program. The program was mostly on distant learning with semi-annual visits to the campus. It was based out of California. There was orientation on the main campus in January. I didn't mind leaving the cold of the Midwest to fly to California. The campus was situated near the ocean. Frequent walks on the beach were wonderful. I attended this Ph.D. program and had the opportunity to meet leaders from around the United States and the world.

Back at home, the organization was proceeding to reorganize and merge the hospital with the clinic. There were new vice president positions opening. I had the credentials to apply. The only thing that was holding me back was the issue of moving further away from direct patient care. Whenever I had to make decisions regarding my professional path, I would talk to God, asking for guidance. I also relied on my colleagues across the country to help me make the decision. The discussions regarding leadership and advancement to the vice president position were helpful and I decided to apply for the vice president position.

Poet David Whyte states, "If you think life is always improving, you're going to miss half of it." I learned that life was cyclical as I walked my path. Every role I started was a crossroad and I would be a novice again, but in a different role. I would work to improve in each role toward becoming an expert. The same process happened as a nurse, student, and leader. Humility and patience are critical along the pathways of life.

Chapter Seven

Traveling and Discovering New Paths

Executive Leadership - Vice President of Regional Services

The interviewing process would start in a week, so I was busy preparing my thoughts on the vice president position and what I could bring to the role. I knew the people interviewing me and felt confident and was able to respond to the questions from both head and heart.

After a few days, I was offered the vice president of regional services. This position covered nineteen counties. There are four small hospitals and thirty-three ambulatory clinics. I did not have any background in ambulatory care and knew I would need to learn a lot.

Every area of care in the reorganization had two vice presidents, a medical vice president and an administrative vice president. The physicians reported to the medical vice president and the administrative directors reported to the administrative vice president. Since these were all new positions, there wasn't an orientation. My medical partner and I were going to have to learn as we went.

I knew the medical vice president. We had worked together when she was a surgical resident in the intensive care unit. That was a relief, and I knew we would work well together. She now was a general surgeon in a rural hospital and clinic. I made my first visit to that site. Most of the clinics and hospitals were about an hour or so from the main campus, which caused me to have a lot of road time. This was a great time to do a lot of thinking and enjoy the countryside. The travel was fine except during the winter months when the roads became slippery.

Rural Patient Care

The small hospitals cared for less acute patients and were similar in how they processed patients. The rural hospitals had an emergency room but did not have an intensive care unit. If patients needed critical care, the emergency room would stabilize the patient and transfer the patient to the main campus. Visiting the nurses and physicians was wonderful. The issues and concerns for them were so different than what I had been accustomed to in a large hospital and clinic.

I listened to stories like this. The nurse shared what it was like to work in a small rural hospital at night. "We truly are on our own. There is no doctor in the hospital and the clinic doctors covered the emergency room if there was need for a physician." She continued to explain what it was like to work in that small hospital. "We have to work as a team. We are always there for the patient and family." She continued, "We are here to give a little one a hug after tears of fear from having a cut sutured.

Or holding a sobbing father in are arms when he had sent his eight-year-old beautiful son to school, only to be called to the emergency room for the death of this same beautiful boy had drowned in the nearby lake because he had tried to cross the lake when the ice gave way."

Another nurse told a story about a first-time mother who showed up at the emergency room. She showed up with a smile on her face, suitcase, and pillow in hand. She and her husband had taken the Lamaze classes and were prepared for the birth of their first baby. The husband parked the car.

The nurse said, "I could tell you she was in full-blown delivery because of the bulge in her pants. The baby's head had already been born and the only thing standing between me and the birth were her stretch pants."

They got the mom in a wheelchair and went to the obstetric department.

The nurse said to the other nurse, "Do you want to take off the stretch pants or catch the baby?"

They didn't even take the mom out of the wheelchair. The nurse directed the mom to lift her butt. She pulled off the stretch pants and the other nurse literally caught the baby! The mom was thrilled, but the dad was a bit disappointed because he wanted to have the full experience.

Another story was about a sick six-year-old, whose mom brought him to the emergency room with a classic case of epiglottitis. The little boy was sweating, drooling, and was in a tripod sitting stance. All signs of epiglottitis. Normally, you would do a lateral neck scan to confirm epiglottitis. Not this time.

The nurse called the doctor and said, "Get in here now. I'll have the ambulance in the bay with a tracheotomy tray in the back of the ambulance. The main hospital is waiting to take the little boy to surgery."

The nurse climbed into the ambulance with the patient and doctor, and they were off. She said they did a lot of praying on the way. They got to the main hospital in forty minutes and the little boy was taken to the operating room within an hour.

There were many stories like these from both the hospital and clinics. Working in rural America is so different than a large city hospital and clinic. The teams in rural settings work with what they have together. The other noticeable difference is that many, if not all, the patients were family and neighbors. They did extraordinary things with limited resources.

I discovered how comfortable I felt with the physicians and staff of the rural facilities. I believe it was because I had been raised on a farm and appreciated the hard work the people were committed to giving no matter what was called for.

I laughed when my medical vice president said to me, "You really understand these people." (Referring to the nurses, support staff, and physicians).

We did an assessment of all the clinics in the nineteen counties. My medical partner and I then gave a report to all the vice presidents, senior vice presidents, and CEO. It was decided that some of the clinics were doing very well. There was one very small clinic that needed to be closed. There were clinics that needed to be remodeled or rebuilt.

Closing and Opening

The small clinic we decided to close was a trailer that had been converted into a clinic. The city had less than 300 people and was thirty miles from another, larger clinic. It seemed appropriate to meet with the staff and city members to let them know. My medical partner and I set up a meeting and drove to the clinic. We knew it would be difficult. The staff and some of the community members were present. We presented the situation and let them know about the closure. The staff wanted to know if they would have jobs. We offered jobs to all the staff at the nearby clinic. The community members were not happy. They said, "This clinic is very important to us. It is as important as our church."

We listened and let them know that we were sorry, but the closure needed to be done. I was learning about how administrative decisions were often very difficult. Some would impact the community, and some would be very political.

The nearby clinic was physically attached to the rural hospital. It needed remodeling. On one side of the hospital was our organization's clinic and on the other side of the hospital was a clinic from another healthcare system. When we met with the rural hospital board, they were less than friendly. I spent time trying to find out why. The CEO and board members were more aligned with the other system's clinic and administration. We were presenting to them a request to expand our clinic, but that would require them to lease more land to us. They firmly refused to approve of the expansion. The staff from our clinic were very concerned that the rural hospital would not let our clinic continue and allow the other system's clinic to take over our clinic. The discussions became very heated. Our senior vice president suggested that our system attorney accompany me to the next board meeting. We drove to the clinic in the evening and once again, the board was very clear that we could not do any expansion. The attorney was not very helpful and spoke in a demeaning manner to the CEO and board members. When we returned to the main campus and gave the executive committee the report of the meeting, our CEO and executives were not happy and looked straight at our system attorney and said, "Guess you were not helpful."

Other comments were made to him, and he stormed out of the meeting. I went back to my office. My secretary came into the office and said the attorney wanted to see me. I went to his office. We had gotten along well before, but he was irate. He was yelling at me about the situation at the rural hospital/clinic. He felt I had set him up. He was calling me nasty things so loudly that the secretaries called the senior vice president and told her what was going on.

Soon, she appeared at the door. She came in, looked at me and said, "You need to leave so I can have a discussion with the attorney."

I went back to my office. Soon the senior vice president was at my door.

She closed the door and said, "I'm so sorry about the attorney. I will not tolerate anyone speaking to a vice president in that manner. He will not be working with us any longer."

I was taken aback. I really didn't expect that this episode would end in a firing. Executive roles have different challenges and situations. I was learning day by day.

At another rural hospital, our clinic was attached to the hospital. It was somewhat the same situation. We wanted to build a new clinic building across from the hospital. This experience went very well. The hospital CEO and community were very happy and supportive. The contracting and business arrangements went well, and we hand groundbreaking for a new clinic building the following spring.

Although there were no more closures, we did some more remodeling and building in the next couple of years. I felt good about all we were accomplishing. I had grown to appreciate our rural clinics, hospitals, and communities.

After three years as vice president of regional services, the senior vice president called me to her office. We meet weekly but this seemed to be a different kind of meeting. She wanted to discuss changing my role. She explained that the current chief nursing officer was not connected to the staff. She also indicated that the executive administration was not pleased with her performance. I knew the chief nursing officer and wondered why she was not successful. The senior vice president asked if I would be willing to be the vice president of nursing, education, and research. I was near completion of my Ph.D. in human and organizational development, and she felt that I would be a good person to lead our nurses, develop an educational campus, and further develop nursing research.

Chapter Eight

Giant Steps

Vice President of Nursing, Education, and Research

It seemed to me after a bit of reflection, this offer was a one-time opportunity and a fitting way to utilize my doctorate degree. I accepted the offer. My office was moved to the research department in the foundation area. Some asked me if I was upset that I would not be in the executive suite. I smiled and responded. I had numerous offices in the past and where they were located never made a difference to me. Once I settled in again, I started the work. I was really excited that I would be able to make rounds in the main hospital and clinic. I started rounding each day to a couple of units, meeting and listening to nurses. I needed to complete a full assessment of nursing at the system level. There seemed a need to let go of the old, which always feels terrible and difficult; before new models and capacity can emerge.

Assessment of Practicing Nurses

The organization had completed an assessment of nursing in the system. I reviewed the material and found many areas that were missing in the assessment. I had been working on my dissertation and decided to move forward with a thorough study. My dissertation was, "Practicing Nurses Perception of Nursing Functions in an Acute and Ambulatory Care Setting: A Secondary Analysis". The original study was a qualitative comparative analysis of thirty-one focus groups conducted in the system during the nursing role redesign project. The project sought nurses and other health care professionals' perceptions of the essential, non-substitutable work of the nurse in the acute and ambulatory settings of healthcare. Each study participant attended a thirty-minute educational session regarding the role redesign project followed by a one and half hour focus group session. The focus groups were voluntary. The original study invited 1,000 nurses and 750 non-nursing healthcare professionals employed full time and part-time in the nineteen counties of the healthcare system. I participated in some of the original focus groups. A total of 172 out of a possible 338 invited nurses and twenty-seven out of a possible seventy-five invited other health care professionals in the system agreed to participate in the original focus groups. The total number of participants was 199.

I went north to an isolated cabin to work on my dissertation research. I brought poster boards, sticky notes, and colored markers. I conducted a thematic content analysis of the thirty-one focus groups. I used a coding method to organize the data into categories and themes.

The total identified parsed statements analyzed were 1022. I wrote down each parsed statement from the nurses and non-nursing participants. Then I started sticking them to the poster boards. I put the statements that were similar in groups. This was an exhausting process. The cabin was situated in the woods, so I periodically went outside to get fresh air and clear my head. After three days of work, I was able to come up with the research questions driven by some key statements. They were notable and I have included some of those statements.

Statements from Nurses

Vital signs are more than just numbers; information is combined with what else is going on with the patient. A nurse knows what to do with the information and recognizes when the patient has a problem. The goal of assessment needs to be more than just technical. The nurse must integrate what he/she sees into what that observation means. Technical assessment is of no value unless there is knowledge of how to act upon that information.

Communication and coordination with all departments is absolutely essential for safe and quality care. This work is about the nurse keeping all the departments and disciplines of the team aware of the patient plan of care and patient needs. We pass on a lot of information to physicians, respiratory therapy, lab, pastoral care. We notify everyone about everything. We are the "go between", often running interference (sic).

Communication of change in status and getting orders from physicians is so important. Physicians use nursing assessments and call back information to determine the next steps for the patient's care. There is a partnership between the nurse and the physician.

Technology requires clinical judgment. Nurses need that judgment and critical thinking to trouble shoot, starting with the patient and working out the systems they are connected to. It is part of our role to collect information but more importantly to interpret data that comes in and synthesize data – kind of like a filter.

Nurses put out fires we don't necessarily start. We are the patient's advocate and need to resolve the concerns of patients and families when there is confusion in messages from physicians and other providers.

One size does not fit all. There must be consideration of specialty. You can't demean the nursing profession to be operational/technical but need to embrace the meaning of the patient interaction. For instance, in the area of assessment, it's more than just technical tasks. It is integrating that they see into what that observation means. Technical assessment is of no value unless there is knowledge of how to act upon the information. One of the strengths of nursing is that it is so diverse. Nurses are intuitive, great listeners and compassionate.

There were many statements that were striking and able to clearly help identify my conceptual framework. This framework led me to lead the nursing practice in the healthcare system.

Contemporary Nursing Practice Implementation

The framework established independent, dependent, and interdependent functions that are exclusive and contribute to practicing contemporary nursing. But at the center of all the nurses' work isthe patient, family, and community. Every element of practice needs to be focused on that core, the patient.

I brought together a team of expert nurses to create a structure that would support the nurses in the organization. The administrative council designed the rest of the nursing councils. The councils decided upon were nursing administrative, nursing education, nursing research (quality), acute care nursing practice, and ambulatory care nursing practice.

The nursing administrative council dealt with policy, procedures, and staffing issues. Participants of the council were clinical nurse managers (head nurses), administrative directors and the vice president of nursing. This ensured that all departments participated in decision making for the whole system.

The nursing education council dealt with nursing

orientation, nursing in-services, and continual education services. Nursing preceptors from every department sat on this council. The work of this council assured us that the system and department education for nurses was consistent and weaved the core values throughout the whole system.

The nursing research council was responsible for quality assurance. The members were nurses who had an interest in research and quality improvement. Performance improvement is a critical element in healthcare. In order to assure quality patient care and to learn from critical incidents of patient care that was not at the level of care expected. Whenever incidents occurred in patient care that was less than optimal, nurses filled our incident reports. The purpose was to review the incidents for trends and to find out where practices broke down. This area is work behind the scenes of excellent patient care. Hospitals and clinics are regulated and overseen by the joint commission of healthcare. This organization makes regular visits to hospitals and clinics to assure quality. This council was key to assuring that the organization was meeting the joint commission standards.

The nursing practice councils for both acute and ambulatory were large councils. They had representatives from each unit or clinic. These councils were critical in assuring that all nurses were represented. They discussed practice, education, and quality issues. The members were key in bringing forth issues the departments and system needed to address. It was a great assurance for front line nurses that their voices mattered in every aspect of patient care.

The nursing structure became a sound system for our organization. At times we made changes to the council structure, but it served the purpose of providing quality care for our patients and each other with passion, dedication, knowledge, engagement, and joy.

Celebration of Nurses

We often don't discuss or emphasis the importance of celebration and just basic fun. Over the years, I have found that when we worked together, we also should take time to play together.

Each department had Christmas parties, birthday celebrations and special event parties. We celebrated Nurses Day and Healthcare Week every year with a system wide celebration. The celebration occurs around May 6th each year. May 6th is Florence Nightingale's birthdate. Nightingale was the founder of nursing.

The celebration was quite elaborate with a great deal of fun and laughter. Its main purpose was to recognize and thank nurses for their hard work and dedication to the patients and families. Two months prior to the celebration we called for nominations of nurses in the areas of administration, education, quality, and practice. The person nominating the nurse wrote letters supporting why this nurse was being nominated. On the evening of the celebration the award winners were able to bring their families to the celebration.

Each year a theme was decided upon to guide the entertainment and decorations. Some of the themes were "The Academy Awards," "The 60s," "Flash Mob," and "A Night with Florence". Not all nurses were able to attend, some had to work. But to ensure they were not left out, food was taken to the departments. Clinics were open during the day, so most nurses could attend the evening celebrations. One year I decided to deliver frozen ice cream desserts to all the regional clinics. I took one of the system vans and drove to all the thirty-three clinics. I started at five o'clock in the morning and got home around 7 PM. I was pretty exhausted by the end of that day but remember the smiles and surprise of the staff in those clinics.

The celebrations were a way for me to check in on the emotional status of our nurses. Were they overall content in their practice? Did they feel they had a voice in operations? I was able to listen to the stories of the nurses who were receiving awards and talk with nurses who were at the celebration.

Even to this day, when I see nurses that worked during this time, they comment on the nursing celebrations. The nurses felt recognized and appreciated.

I always sent a message at the holidays. We published a nursing new letter monthly, so this was an excellent tool to get a message out to each and every nurse. Here is an example.

Thanksgiving Message from the Chief Nursing Officer

I can hardly believe another year is almost gone. Gone, but it will never be forgotten. Over the next few weeks, I suggest you spend some time thinking about all we have accomplished and all that we need to be grateful for. I thought I could help you by putting my "thank" list in front of you.

First, I am thankful for the great spiritual energy that surrounds me, each and every day. The energy I am blessed with from nature, my friends, my family, my colleagues, and community. I am especially thankful for you. Each and every one of you!

You have surpassed any of my dreams by delivering the highest of quality, safe care to our patients and families. This was demonstrated by the joint commission offering no recommendations for the nursing staff at our system. I have worked as a nurse for thirty years and have experienced many joint commission visits. We have never had such an outstanding report. Thank you!

I am thankful for those of you who push me to speed up and those of you who encourage me to slow down.

Somewhere in the middle of fast and slow is solace and peace. I am grateful for those of you who offer a smile and warm hello as you pass me and others every day. I thank you for times you make me laugh and times when you make me cry.

I am thankful for our leaders who spend endless days and nights trying to light the way to the future even though there are many hills and mountains to climb. They give me strength and hope to go on and discover a new way and a new day.

Personally, I am grateful that I do not have to walk seven miles to the nearest clinic in the cold and wind to seek help for my swollen feet and legs because that is the only health care facility in a thirty-mile radius. I am grateful that when I come home, I can turn on lights, take a hot bath, and sink into a warm bed. Many people have none of that. I wonder why I am blessed, and they are not. But perhaps they are the ones that are blessed. I am so grateful for all of us who reach out to hold the hands of the dying and the hands of those who are left behind.

I am thankful to each one of you who see your colleague in stress and fear and reach out to let them know they will be OK. One of my dear colleagues gave me a message that I read every morning and would like to share with you.

"Don't worry, you'll be OK. Slowing down is good. Wisdom simmers and steeps and grows with time. Stop pushing yourself. You are enough just as you are. There is no need to perform. Just relax and let life unfold. You have what it takes to handle anything. Good and great things come from patience, not pushing. Let space and time reveal something miraculous. Trust life: accept where you are right now. Stop the judgment of yourself and others".

Have a Blessed and Happy Thanksgiving!

Western Campus Nursing Program

One of the many expectations in my role as vice president of nursing, education, and research was to explore the possibility of opening a nursing program in our healthcare system. We already had a medical residency program aligned with a large university system in the state. I went to that system to discuss the possibility of creating a western campus on our campus. I was delighted to discover that the dean of nursing at the university was excited to work on the creation of a western campus of nursing.

We had several nurses who had their master's degree in nursing and would be able to become instructors on the western campus. Since I hold a Ph.D., I would be able to meet the requirements of an assistant dean. The students spent their first two years on the main university campus and the last two years on our western campus.

The curriculum was developed by the university and our faculty taught academic and clinical classes on our campus.

Our first year was a bit bumpy but at the end of two years we graduated five nurses. Doesn't sound like many, but some of those nurses decided to start their nursing career with us. We increased the enrollment each year until we graduated ten nurses. It was a great experience for all who were involved with the program. The program lasted several years. The program cost and difficulty recruiting faculty led to the closure.

Nursing Research

Under the large department of research, there was a small group of nurses who worked with physicians to do medical research studies. This was a very unique role for nurses. The nurses would meet with patients to see if they qualified for a specific study and then if the patients did meet the requirements, the nurses would give the experimental medications or treatments.

When I worked with this group, I decided to develop an area for nursing scientists to bring their studies to this department. There were a few nursing scientists who worked with nursing staff who were doing research in the area of nursing. The work brought forth new nursing practice to improve patient care.

After several years as vice president of nursing practice, education and research, the senior vice president called me to her office. I always knew when she was going to present a new path or experience. I wasn't wrong about the new path but was very surprised.

She said, "Have you ever thought about being a dean of nursing?"

I said, "I am the assistant dean for western campus."

"I know that," she said. "I meant a nursing dean for a full nursing program," she continued.

"What are you talking about?" I said.

She looked at me with a smile and said, "The president of the university across town met with me and was wondering if you would be interested an interim dean position?"

I was shocked. I only had experience in nursing education with the western campus. I had taught a few classes in the master's program, but I really didn't think I had the experience required to be a full-time dean.

The senior vice president said, "I know you don't think you have the experience, but it wouldn't be the first role you took on without a lot of experience. The least you can do is meet with the university president."

"I guess I can do that," I said. "What about my full time as vice president of nursing practice, education and research here?"

"Well, let's take one step at a time. For now, maybe you could keep nursing research," she said.

As I reflected on this opportunity that evening, I

thought about all my steps and paths in nursing. Perhaps this was another path to take. I set up a meeting with the university president the next day.

Chapter Nine

Unlikely Steps

Dean of Nursing

I met with the president of the university. I knew him from meetings and alumni celebrations. This university was where I went to school for my bachelor in nursing. His office was a large, beautiful office. His secretary was warm and greeted me with a hot cup of coffee and escorted me into the president's office.

We started the conversation with some cordial small talk.

Then he said, "I talked to your boss about the possibility of becoming our interim dean of nursing."

I nodded.

"You may wonder why," he continued.

"Yes, it seems strange to me since I do not have formal background as a full-time professor. My only work with academia has been with the western campus," I responded.

"I know about your background and credentials and that is exactly why I asked if you would meet with me," he said. "You see, I don't need the person in this role as a professor, past dean, or someone who has worked in academia. What I need is a nurse leader who can assess, plan, implement, and develop our nursing program for the future. I'm looking for someone that knows nursing in acute care, ambulatory care, education, and research. You fit the need, perfectly," he said.

After an hour of discussion, I said I needed to think and pray about it. I said I would let him know in a couple of days.

The first director of nursing I worked for was a Franciscan sister and now was in the Franciscan nursing home. I decided to go see her and get her advice. The nursing home is located out in the country with a view of beautiful woodlands. We sat outside on the deck facing the woodland. After we chatted for a while, I told her that I had been offered to become interim dean at the university. She was quiet and I waited for her response.

She smiled and looked at me. She said, "You know I can't believe what you have done since you were a new graduate. I still remember our lunch before you took the head nurse job at the Lutheran hospital. I really did not believe you would become so successful. But here you are with a Ph.D. and being asked to be a dean. Of course, you should take this opportunity. Just think how many faculty and students you can inspire."

She grabbed my hands and we hugged. I will always remember that moment. I decided to accept the challenge. I would become the interim dean of nursing at the university.

I kept my office at the healthcare system as head of

nursing research and packed up some of the things I would need in my office at the university. This new pathway seemed like becoming a novice once again. The environment, work, and people were new. I did know many of the nursing faculty from my previous work and organizations. Faculty and other deans I would get to know and appreciate.

In every transition, you bring with you experiences and knowledge from previous work. I had many tools in my leadership toolbox that would be helpful as I started this new path. The first steps are always hard. But I knew I was being guided by a greater power and trusted that he would be at my side.

Assessment – Know the condition of the flock.

I went back to my article, "Leading Nurses Like a Shepherd," to put my go forward plan together. The first thing was to get to know the flock. Many of the nursing faculty were colleagues I knew from nursing organizations and other work. Some of the nursing faculty, I did not know. I decided to meet with each individual faculty and ask them three basic questions:

What is your background?

What are your goals and dreams?

What do you expect of me as your Interim Dean of Nursing?

These were the same questions I had asked of the first staff I had as a manager.

There were thirty nursing faculty and a few administrative assistants. Each session was thirty minutes long. I learned quickly that some of the faculty were open and wanted to share. Others were quiet and almost cold toward me. Still, I greeted them with open arms. They all called me, "Dr. Gerke." I never made people address me as "doctor," but in this environment, titles were extremely important. I became aware of the importance of calling them "professor" or "associate professor".

Some of the professors did not feel I should be in this position. I wanted to understand this attitude and what was driving them to have these feelings. I learned that the previous dean had been asked to step down and many felt that the president and vice president had done this without due process.

I meet with the president weekly for a month and discovered the rationale for his decision. I asked if he had shared his concerns with the dean and faculty.

He said, "Somewhat, but they were too hostile to really get into the deep conversations required."

He and the board wanted to expand the nursing program by adding more students and to admit two-year nurses into the program without having them repeat the first two years. I wanted to open that Pandora's box.

I said, "With the increased demand for nurses, this

makes good sense. I need to hear from the faculty what all their concerns are about expanding the program. I need to listen to them and gain their trust."

The first faculty meeting was telling. The assistant dean and I sat at a table in front of tables filled with faculty members. The secretary sat at a side table and took minutes. The assistant dean introduced me and led the meeting. The meeting was reports from various committees. There wasn't any discussion. At the end, the assistant dean asked if I would like to say a few words.

I took a deep breath and said, "Thank you all for taking time to meet with me in our one-on-one discussions. I know that you are not excited about me being your interim dean. I understand. I do not have an academic background. But I have a leadership background. What I ask of you is to help me, help you and the nursing program. What do you see as the major issues or problems we need to work on?"

There was silence. I waited.

Finally, one faculty member raised their hand and I nodded, and she said, "We do not have enough faculty."

I said, "Could you explain to me how you determine the number of faculty you need?"

She responded, "We base it on the number of students to faculty ratio. It is the number of classes we have to teach and the clinical experiences we have to supervise."

I looked directly at the faculty and said, "Are there a

few of you who would be willing to sit down with me, the assistant dean, and secretary to put together a document with exact numbers and cost of the ideal faculty number? I am willing to bring that information forward to the vice president and president."

There were three faculty members who volunteered, and I asked the secretary to set up a few meetings.

I ended the meeting by saying, "We will present the document to all of you at the next faculty meeting before I take the proposal to the vice president. It is getting late; I know you would like to go home. I will end with this for you to think about. We need to let go of the old and I know how terrible that feels. But we have to let it go before new life and capacity can arise. I am a leader whose door is always open. Feel free to stop by anytime."

The first six months of being the interim dead was like swimming against the current of a deep river. I learned that the faculty needed a lot of love and recognition. So, I would eat lunch with them as often as I could. I attended one class of each faculty and wrote a summary of my evaluation of the class and then met with them. This was time-consuming but worth it. I learned a great amount about the faculty and the program.

I learned about how faculty became tenured. It is quite a process. There are total books on the subject. There is a whole system of how the faculty can achieve tenure. What they must do each year, leading up to becoming tenured. I usually takes five years to become tenure. I wondered why being tenure was so important. Tenure promotes stability, increases pay, and gives recognition to faculty. My background in staff performance evaluations helped me with this process. There were some faculty who were approaching being tenured and they had to put together a lengthy paper explaining how they met all the various tenants of being tenured. Once they had completed the packet, they were presented to a university wide committee.

I also was interim dean of the social work program, dietetics program and master of mental health program. These areas were smaller, but I use the same template as I had with the nursing program. I met with each faculty member, attended their faculty meetings, and attended at least one of their classes.

After the first semester, I felt that I was getting more organized and developing a routine. It was great to have a few weeks off to just get caught up with family, relax, and reflect.

The vice president and president of the university were willing to invest in more faculty, but they also wanted to increase the enrollment. I knew this was not going to be easy, but that was why I had taken the position. During the second semester, I felt I could start making some changes. I interviewed for new nursing faculty, of course a faculty committee interviewed the candidates as well.

There wasn't a big pool of candidates but at least we were able to bring on a few for the following fall semester. It helped that I knew the healthcare organizations and could recruit nurses to become faculty members.

I wanted to be more present with the nursing students. The faculty really didn't understand why I wanted to do that; they felt they were the connection to the students. I wanted to hear from the students to find out if we were meeting their expectations. I wanted to know if they had ideas for changes that would make the program stronger. I started "Fireside Chats with the Dean". I held monthly sessions, open to all nursing students in the lobby of the nursing center by the fireplace. At first, not many students showed up. But eventually more students came. I really enjoyed listening to their stories and ideas.

There are many ceremonies and celebrations in academia. Graduation of course is the main event and takes a great deal of planning. The nursing program was the largest program and had a pinning ceremony for students entering into their third year as well as the graduation ceremony. The ceremonies were held in the campus auditorium with parents and friends in the audience. I gave my speeches for the pinning ceremony. My focus was the students, but I also gave recognition to the families and friends who supported the students on their educational journey.

During the summer, I was able to get a great deal of work done. There were only the deans, vice president, and president on campus along with administrative assistants and other staff. During those months we were able to do strategic planning and work on the next academic year.

Implementing Change – The Staff of Direction

I was ready for the second year. The fall brought the students and faculty back. Every fall, the dean spoke to the students. I used this opportunity to talk about the soul of nursing and how they needed to understand the honor of being a nurse. The wheels of change go slowly. I was now ready to present to the faculty the proposal to change the nursing program to dual enrollment. This would mean that the program would admit students twice a year. One starting in first semester and another enrollment starting in second semester. We averaged an enrollment of 100 students. By initiating dual enrollment, we would increase the enrollment to 180 students. There was a great deal of work to accomplish this change. The recruitment and admission department, the class scheduling, clinical experience scheduling, pinning, and graduation ceremonies. But the greatest hurdle was faculty scheduling. I took the remainder of the year to accomplish the work. Over two years we added eight faculty. The additional faculty could accommodate the additional students.

Need for Transitions – The Rod of Correction

There were some faculty who could not and would not accept any changes. A few were nearing the end of their career. I spent time with each of them to listen and offer my opinion of their options. Sometimes, I have learned, people need to be freed up to explore other opportunities. Others need someone to blame their inability to change on someone. Leaving staff go is hard. Over my career, it never got easier. So, with the need for more faculty, and turnover of faculty, the situation became even harder. The faculty who decided to leave were tenured, so the departure was on them to make the final decision. Three faculty decided to leave for the next year. Again, we started recruitment of new faculty. It was just part of the work.

There also were some students who were unable to stay in the program. The nursing program is rigorous, there are general education courses like biology, chemistry, physiology, and history. But these courses are much more difficult than the same courses in high school. When the faculty monitored the students, they coached the students. However, sometimes the students were not a match for the program. At times, I met with a student and usually they brought their parents with them. On one occasion a faculty came to me and said one of the nursing students was failing and wondered if I would meet with the student and her parents. I invited the student and parents into my office. I listened to their perspective.

The student said, "I know I am not doing well in the program, but I would like to keep trying."

The father interrupted and said, "My wife and I are both nurses and can't understand why our daughter is struggling in this nursing program. She was an excellent student in high school."

After they presented their perspectives, I said, "I think we have two issues. First, college curriculum and study are very different and more rigorous than high school." I looked straight at the student and continued, "Second, the student needs to make sure he or she wants to be a nurse. Mary, I see you are exceeding in biology, do you want to be a nurse?" I asked.

She was quiet, a tear ran down her cheek. Mary said, "I really want to be a biologist, but my parents want me to be a nurse."

Her parents were a bit shocked. They had assumed Mary wanted to be a nurse, like them.

I said, "There is great need for biologists in healthcare, and many other fields. Would you and your parents like to meet with the department head of biology? He would be able to discuss all the options and opportunities there are in the field of biology."

They agreed and Mary was transferred to biology as her major.

There were other student–parent miscommunications. I learned to encourage parents to explore the question as to what the child wants and needs versus what the parent wants and needs. I decided to weave this learning into the freshman orientation.

I completed the second year. I met with the president of the university and senior vice president of the health system, and we all decided it would be best if I left the healthcare system completely and focus on the work of dean. It was too hard to maintain a presence in nursing research at the healthcare system and do the work of dean at the university.

Completely leaving the healthcare organization I had spent thirty-seven years of my life in was filled with mixed emotions. I have so many memories and wonderful friends from those thirty-seven years. I knew it was time to hand the reigns over to the next generation of nurses and leaders.

I remained at the university for a third year. The third year was consumed with several initiatives we had started. First launching the dual enrollment. The community was thrilled to have the university bring on more nursing students. The enrollment in fall remained the same, around 120 students. The enrollment for January semester was around seventy students. The faculty had increased but there were bumps in the road that we dealt with one by one.

The second initiative was going through the accreditation process. This work fell on a few faculty members, the administrative assistant and me. I had gone through a similar process at the healthcare system. The accrediting agency's purpose is to assure that the organizations are meeting the standards to assure quality. In this case, the quality of nursing education. All areas are evaluated. Faculty credentials, curriculum plans for all courses, financial integrity, and operation of the program. We had worked on preparation for a site visit for a year. The surveyors came and were pleased with the work of this nursing program. At the end of the process, the nursing program was accredited for ten years. This is the highest accreditation, and everyone was very pleased with the outcome.

The third initiative was pursuing a grant for a few million dollars over five years to recruit underprivileged students. The university is centered in a city surrounded by rural and small communities. We visited many of the same hospitals, clinics, and schools, I had visited as the vice president of the region. It was really fun to meet with people from the past and they welcomed us with open arms. Writing a grant is very difficult and I was lucky to have a great grant writer to complete the application. The grant was approved. Two faculty and one administrative assistant work was adjusted to manage the grant. Events were held in high schools to recruit students. The grant paid for the students' tuition and room and board. The first year brought in eight students. The work was well worth the effort for the university and the students.

Late in fall of the third year, the vice president invited me to apply for the permanent dean position. One of my mentors from the past shared the wisdom of knowing when to leave. Knowing when to leave takes praying and meditating on what is good for the organization and what is good for you. After several days, I knew that God was directing me to move on and I decided that it was time for me to retire. I knew that I had met the expectations the university had asked of me. Of course, there still was a lot of work to do but I felt a new dean who had the experience and energy to take the program to the next level was the best thing for the nursing program.

I wasn't part of the recruiting of a new dean. The candidates seemed well qualified and by spring a new dean had been selected to start after graduation. I decided to work with the new dean to ensure she had an orientation and transition I had not received. I reviewed with her each faculty member's performance and where they were in the tenure process. I went through each initiative we had accomplished in three years. It was good for the new dean, but it also was good for me as I looked to the next step, retirement.

The last few days on campus, I packed up my belongings and made visits to people I had gotten to know on campus to say goodbye. Leaving the university wasn't quite as difficult as leaving the healthcare facility but it still was another goodbye. I looked forward to the next steps and adventures.

Chapter Ten

Muses

Retirement – Into the Woods

On June 30, I left the university and headed to my cabin in northern Wisconsin. The process of retirement takes quiet time and meditation. It was strange not to have a schedule, meetings, and appointments. I immersed myself in nature. What a great gift to be silent and listen to the call of nature. I'm sure not all people have this opportunity, and I am so grateful. It also was a time to really have deep conversations with the creator. I started seeing nature as I never had before. It made me feel closer to God. I was so impressed at his power and glory. The spirit of God is deeply rooted in every creature. The sunsets and sunrises were beautiful, and I appreciate them so much more than I ever had in the past.

For the first few years I was able to work on the property and busy myself with gardening, reading, woodworking and crafts. It was so fulfilling to tap into a creative side of me I never had time to do.

I had packed up all my past writings and memories of years of working in the profession of nursing. I decided it was time to go through all the boxes, books, and documents. I realized that there were definite themes throughout my career. There also were things I needed to let go of and throw away.

Many of the themes and memories I have shared in this book.

Principles and Themes of My Journey

I learned the importance to listen to God and people who brought a message from God as to what needed to be done or said in every step of the way. When I was at a lost for words, I just trusted that God would give me words to say. At times I was shocked at the words that came out of my mouth. Completely surrendering to God is not easy because we think we know what needs to be done. However, if we have trust and faith that the will of God will be done, life can be a lot less stressful. I know this is not always easy but its worth trying to let God lead the way.

The patient and family always came first. In every role, I always did or asked what was in the best interest of the patient and family. My actions and decisions were based on that principle.

Doing things differently was usually a good thing, even though it was hard and not always pleasing to others. There are reasons to hold on to things. Science for example develops knowledge through research that helps guide us and improve our understanding of our environment, minds, and bodies. The learnings that protect us rarely change. But there are reasons to change. When new ideas and experiences encourage us to take a new or different process. As I learned, if you don't try new ways of doing things, you will never know if there are better ways to do things. I became a risk taker and that was a blessing and at times a curse.

When leading people you must walk in their footsteps and work side-by-side with them. Sometimes leading by example was the best and strongest way to lead. I learned how important it was to have compassion and empathy for each and every person that came into my life. I started asking myself why people came into my life. Sometimes I did not know right away but if I was patient, I found out why they came into my life. All people behave the way they do for a reason. Often, they do not tell you why. So, it is better, I believe, to just know there is a reason and not judge them.

I learned to lean on others when the going gets tough. I always was blessed to have family, friends and colleagues who were there to walk through the storm with me. I learned to be able to ask for guidance and help with issues and problems. There were always people who were willing to be there in good and hard times.

I learned to trust my instincts. Most of the time my instincts were right but there were times when they led me down the wrong path. I also learned and continued to learn that when things go wrong you have to forgive yourself and let it go. This might be hard to do but the weight of worrying about them just adds to stress and confusion. The next day comes, and new opportunities emerge.

Throughout my career and life experience, I often wasn't very patient. I expected the outcome to happen right away. I think I have learned that patience is a good policy and should be in everyone's toolbox of life. I have to admit I still work on practicing patience every day. Many folks have said, "What will be, will be. Trust when the time is right the outcome will present itself."

Being a novice is not a one-time deal. From a novice to expert happens at every step of career and life.

Finally, life is a journey, one step at a time. There are good times and bad times, but each moment is part of the journey. Learning from mistakes enriches the future and celebrating the good times brings joy to the soul.

Conclusion – A Time for Everything

Ecclesiastes 3:1-8 (International Version) There is a time for everything and a season for every activity under the heaven:

A time to be born and a time to die,
A time to plant and time to uproot,
A time to kill and a time to heal,
A time to tear down and a time to build,
A time to weep and a time to laugh,
A time to mourn and a time to dance,
A time to scatter stones and a time to gather them,
A time to embrace and a time to give up,
A time to keep and a time to throw away,
A time to tear and a time to mend,
A time to be silent and a time to speak,
A time to love and a time to hate,
A time for war and a time for peace.

Resources

Leman K, Pentak W. *The Way of the Shephard*. Grand Rapids, MI: Zondervan: 2004.

Henry, Linda Gambee & James Douglas. *The Soul of the Caring Nurse*. Washington, DC: American Nurses Association: 2004.

The Great Adventure, Your Journey Through the Bible. (2001). Ascension. West Chester, Pennsylvania

Tye, Joe. *The Florence Prescription*. Studio 6 Sense: 2009.

Williamson, Marianne. *A Return to Love*. HarperCollins: 1996.

Biographical Sketch

Mary Lu Gerke is retired. During her 41-year career in nursing, she held the following roles: medical and critical care practicing nurse, Clinical Educator, head nurse, Administrative Director, Vice President of Regional Services, Vice President of Nursing, Education and Research. She served as Interim Dean of Nursing, Graduate Nursing DNP, Social Work, Nutrition/Dietetics, Psychology, Criminal Justice, and Master of Mental Health Counseling.

Education includes:

BSN from Viterbo College, La Crosse, Wisconsin in 1974

Master's degree in nursing administration from Winona State University, Minnesota in 1975

Master's degree in human and organizational development from Fielding University, Santa Barbara, California in 2000,

Ph.D. in human and organizational development from Fielding University, Santa Barbara, California in 2005

Gerke focused on nursing, organizational leadership and development, research, ethics, conflict engagement, innovation and change, generational diversity, conflict engagement and legislative issues in healthcare.

She has given presentations on leadership, generational diversity, conflict, humor, nursing, and storytelling nationally and internationally. She has published in nursing books and journals.

Passionate about risk and change, Gerke led innovative projects like the Clinical Nurse Leader role at Gundersen Health System as well as Role Identification and Conflict Engagement creating a Healing Environment. She worked with Dr. Jean Watson and Robert Browning in integrating Caritas with Heart Math at Gundersen Health System, La Crosse, Wisconsin.

She ended her professional career at Viterbo University, La Crosse, Wisconsin. As Interim Dean of Nursing she led the program to start dual enrollment, increasing enrollment from 100 to 180 students. The nursing program was awarded a grant to recruit nursing students from underserved areas of Wisconsin.

Printed in the USA
CPSIA information can be obtained
at www.ICGtesting.com
LVHW010752110524
779587LV00015BA/887

9 798890 272881